PERFECT HEALTH
The Natural Way

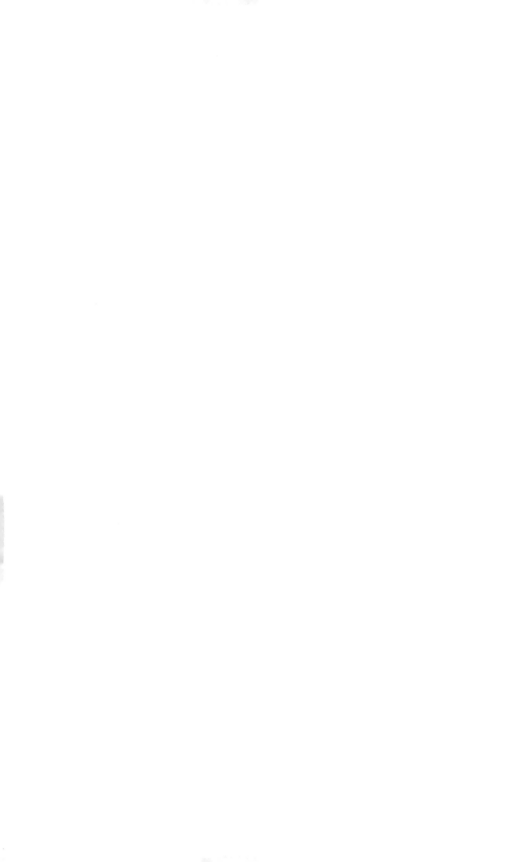

Praise for Mary-Ann Shearer and Perfect Health

As a medical practitioner, I can think of no finer way to enrich a person's life than to improve and ultimately maximize his or her state of health. *Perfect Health* is a clear, interesting, and well-researched introduction to the principles of an optimum lifestyle. Having incorporated them into my own life and the daily lives of my family, friends, and patients, the rewards and benefits have been immeasurable.

—LEIGH SINDELMAN, PH.D.

Perfect Health is a book aimed simply at improving long-term family and individual health. The dedication of the author in sharing her research of the optimal eating plan is unsurpassed, and the passion she feels with regard to this all-important subject is tangible. Her references are both sound and current. I have found this book to be a valuable tool both in my own research and as a reference for my family's well-being.

—CHARLOTTE MESCHEDE
B.Sc. Dietetics (University of Natal), South Africa

The demands of our modern lifestyle cause significant detrimental effects on eyes and vision, such as dry eyes, spiraling prescriptions, unsightly and uncomfortable conjunctival degenerations, cataracts, and retinal deterioration. Having personally enjoyed the benefits of the Perfect Health lifestyle, it is wonderful to be able to make lifestyle recommendations that could reverse the deterioration, rather than just mask the symptoms.

Perfect Health is just so logical. It has ensured supreme health through the "character-forming" times we have survived over the years. Thank you, Mary-Ann and Mark, for persevering to share this with any who would listen.

—GORDON BURNHAM-KING
Optometrist, Former President, South African Optometric Association

Eating the Natural Way has improved my energy levels and made me a calmer person. As a consequence, I am able to cope very well in stressful conditions. Many people look for solutions when they encounter problems in their lives. We are fortunate and very happy that we have found Perfect Health while we are still young. It has improved our lives tremendously and we hope to grow old gracefully.

—ALISON MENDES
Natural Health Consultant, U.K.

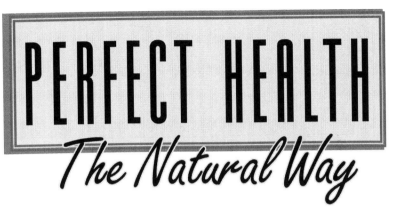

The Natural Way

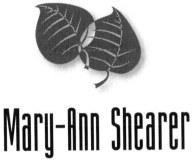

Mary-Ann Shearer

BenBella

BENBELLA BOOKS, INC.

Dallas, Texas

BenBella Books, Inc.
10300 N. Central Expressway, Suite 400
Dallas, TX 75231
www.benbellabooks.com
Send feedback to feedback@benbellabooks.com

Proofreading by Emily Chauviere, Anjali Lahiri, and Yara Abuata
Cover design by Allison Bard
Mary-Ann Shearer cover photo © Studio Toselli
Text design and composition by John Reinhardt Book Design
Printed in the United States of America

Library of Congress Cataloging-in-Publication Data

Shearer, Mary-Ann.
    Perfect health : the natural way / Mary-Ann Shearer.—1st BenBella books ed.
    p. cm.
    ISBN 1-933771-08-9
    1. Raw foods. 2. Nutrition. 3. Health. I. Title.

TX392.S54 2006
641.5'63—dc22

                                                                  2006039328

Distributed by Perseus Distribution
(www.perseusdistribution.com)
To place orders through Perseus Distribution:
Tel: 800-343-4499
Fax: 800-351-5073
E-mail: orderentry@perseusbooks.com

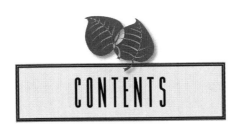

CONTENTS

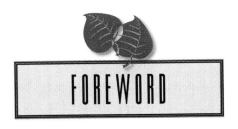

FOREWORD

MY FIRST HEALTH BOOK, *The Natural Way,* was released in October 1991 in South Africa. The book took off and is, to date, the bestselling health and nutrition book in southern Africa. Just months before my final draft went to the publisher I discovered that the most comprehensive research to be done in the field had just been completed. Then, in 2005 Dr. T. Colin Campbell's epic book *The China Study* was released in the U.S. This book had been written by the head of the study. What is exciting for me, and other people who have reaped the benefits of *The Natural Way,* is that his research completely supports the lifestyle *The Natural Way* promotes.

In this new edition, *Perfect Health: The Natural Way,* especially written for the U.S., I have added more information to help you take responsibility for your health. It seems bizarre that when I first wrote *The Natural Way,* I did it by hand (I could not type well in those days—a mere fifteen years ago), and there were no cell phones or e-mail, and a laptop, like the one I am typing this on, was something I only dreamt of!

I now have a Web site—www.mary-anns.com—and a free e-mail newsletter that goes out every two weeks to people across the world, a monthly Digimag, or digital magazine, on DVD that includes cooking demonstrations, interviews, seminars and talks, and trained Natural Health consultants and coaches. It makes it much easier to offer you nutritional and lifestyle support. Although just reading this book is enough to revolutionize the health of thousands with no additional help. Many of their success stories are told in this updated version.

I have also penned five other titles, which are available on our Web site. The demand *The Natural Way* created has resulted in my husband, Mark, and I developing a range of healthy food products under Mary-Ann's label. A Natural Health and Nutrition Course and a Natural Health Consulting Course were established to help many of you who want to assist others. (See www.mary-anns.com.)

Health has become mainstream and it is awesome to see how families across the world are hungry for real knowledge and wisdom about health without the hype and sales pitches. People have taken responsibility for their health and well-being, and gone on to help others do the same.

Writing this book has been one of the most rewarding things we could have done. Mark and I are constantly blown away by the testimonies we have heard. There is nothing better than seeing people literally change before our eyes.

Weight drops off, sinuses clear up, hair begins to grow thick and glossy; sleeping problems, tonsillitis, painful periods, cancer, heart disease, diabetes, high blood pressure, ME (Myalgic Encephalomyelitis, also known as Yuppie Flu), lupus, digestive problems, and even AIDS symptoms disappear and are replaced with glowing health and energy. People report that their brains appear to be functioning properly for the first time and marriages and relationships drastically improve. (I know ours did.)

Does this happen overnight? No. It is a long-term commitment to a healthy lifestyle with no gimmicks or false promises.

Anyone can follow these principles; no matter what age or income group they fall in, the Perfect Health principles are universal and simple enough for anyone to understand and implement.

It is all about understanding how your body works and learning to listen to your body.

By committing to the Perfect Health lifestyle, you will find, as thousands of other people have, that you can:

- Eliminate and prevent disease
- Reach and maintain your ideal weight
- Have increased energy
- Sleep better
- Have regular bowel movements
- Take control of your health habits

- Improve brain function, moods, behavior, and concentration
- Have positive emotions and outlook on life
- Improve your self-esteem, and have more time and energy to focus on loved ones
- Find it easier to attain your goals and dreams
- Live a longer and more enriching life

"To Health!"
—Mary-Ann, *2007*

CHAPTER ONE

The Shearer Family
How Our Diet and Health Evolved

WHY HAVE I WRITTEN THIS BOOK? There are many reasons.

I first became interested in nutrition in my late teens. I wanted to take charge of my own health. Perhaps this sounds pretentious, but when I looked at animals in the wild and compared them with domesticated animals, I began to realize that diet and lifestyle play a major role in attaining health and well-being. Have you ever seen or heard of an over-weight buck or deer suffering from gout, ear infections, or osteoporosis? Neither have I. Have you ever encountered a domesticated cat or dog suffering from these ailments? I have, too!

In my search, I read just about every health book and article I could get my hands on. The result? Total confusion! And what's more, I was branded a "health nut." There I was, drinking apple cider, vinegar, and honey to start my day, followed by my own homemade muesli with my own homemade yogurt and unheated natural honey. I would mostly drink herbal teas, an occasional cup of Ceylon tea and, very rarely, a cup of decaffeinated coffee. This was followed by lunch, usually my own homemade bread with light margarine, even lighter cottage cheese, and a still lighter health salt. Perhaps I'd have a slice of tomato or some lettuce for variety. And I'd always take vitamins after a meal: calcium for healthy bones, vitamin A for skin and eyes, vitamin B (complex, of course) for pre-menstrual tension, hair, and nails, vitamin C for colds and flu, and many more. Supper would consist of vegetables with unpolished rice (naturally), and fish, chicken, or red meat limited to two or three times a week—a very balanced diet according to most dieticians.

So what was wrong? I should have been happy and healthy; after all, I was at my thinnest ever, having been on countless diets over the years to rid myself of my pear-shaped body, and I thought I had finally found the way to live. The problem was that despite my rigorous "health" regime, I was far from well.

As a child I had to cope with the normal childhood ailments, and the only problem I seemed repeatedly to have was that fever blisters kept appearing with irritating regularity. (I have since discovered that whenever I eat anything containing egg, this reaction is triggered.) The first health problem I encountered in adulthood was recurring indigestion—this surfaced after I had been married for a couple of years. Mark also suffered from this problem even though we ate relatively basic foods. In fact, when I married him he was the biggest junk-food eater I had ever met; he practically lived on burgers, fries, coffee, and sodas. Then we began eating a healthy diet (or at least our understanding of healthy) and he still had health problems and no energy even though his diet improved.

Then I started having problems with my hands. I developed severe dermatitis between my fingers and on my palms. At this stage I thought I had merely inherited the problem from my mother—who suffered from dermatitis, as well—and followed the same route she did—to the doctor. He, after taking one look at my hands, prescribed the same cream that my mother used, which, not surprisingly, did the same as it had for her—absolutely nothing!

Then I followed the "guinea-pig" stage of the treatment. Various creams, including cortisone-based products, were applied to the affected area, but to no avail. I was then told not to let my hands ever get sweaty. I stopped putting soap of any kind on my skin. (To this day Mark still washes the dishes—one of the many reasons we are still happily married thirty years later!) But none of these precautions made any difference in my condition.

After three or four years of battling and hiding my hands from view, a third health problem manifested itself: I began sneezing. Not just an occasional sneeze, but continual sneezing accompanied by an ever-streaming nose. The only time my nose wasn't running was when it was blocked. Can you imagine my frustration? After all, I was so health-conscious! In fact, I became the family joke: "Why don't you eat burgers with us, then you'll be as healthy as we are," they taunted. Off I traipsed to the doctor again. This time various nasal sprays were prescribed and heat treatment was provided by a physiotherapist. This cleared my nose for an hour or two. Then the symptoms came back—with a vengeance!

Perhaps you think I'm exaggerating, but my problem was so severe that I couldn't sleep properly at night. And I was keeping Mark awake, too. I then became pregnant with my third daughter, and I was concerned about the possible effects that all the medication I'd been taking would have on my unborn child. I then took myself to a naturopath/homoeopath.

I was very impressed! She spent nearly an hour asking me about my circumstances—where I grew up, what type of background I came from, what type of marriage I had. She told me that if I weren't a happily married and content woman, I would be extremely ill. She declared my constitution to be very sensitive. I would, therefore, have to stop eating the foods of the deadly nightshade family: tomatoes, potatoes, eggplants (also known as aubergine or brinjal), and green bell peppers. I also had to swallow a series of powders. I followed all these instructions to the letter. The result? No improvement whatsoever! I was then instructed to cut out pineapples and bananas, but this still left me sneezing and scratching my hands and very disillusioned. Next was a naturopath who gave me a box full of vitamins. I was already taking a lot so what difference would more make? Well, exactly nothing. In fact, I seemed to get worse.

Then one Sunday while Mark was reading the paper, he came across a book review on *Food Combining for Health*. Apparently, this was the book to get if you suffered from allergies of any description. I was a bit skeptical after all my failed experiments, but Mark suggested I give it a try. What did I have to lose? I was encouraged by the fact that this time there were no drugs, powders, or pills, and I could eat all the foods I had cut out from my diet under instruction from the naturopath/homoeopath. All I had to ensure was that I did not eat complex carbohydrates with concentrated protein (refer to page 265 and chapter four). Although it sounded rather strange, the reasoning made sense.

The results were unbelievable: I stopped sneezing immediately, and four days later my hands were totally clear. But ever skeptical, I thought, *Let's see how long this lasts.*

The indigestion stopped and two weeks later my many symptoms had not returned. After two months I thought I was totally cured and returned to my old eating habits. The morning after I had eaten a normal supper, I woke up with a streaming nose and noticed the little tell-tale blisters between my fingers. *This had to be a coincidence*, I told myself. How could I live without lasagna (meat and pasta) for the rest of my life? Needless to say, the indigestion returned, the dermatitis flourished, and the sneezing continued. The solution was unavoidable. I had to change my lifestyle and my way of eating. Mark was very supportive as he, too, wanted to be rid of his indigestion and exhaustion, and he agreed to change with me, and so the whole family changed. In next to no time all our troublesome symptoms disappeared. Not only were we completely well, but we both had considerably more energy.

By this stage our friends and family had written us off as complete health freaks, and when my daughters had health problems—Melissa got tonsillitis and Marie-Claire's nose streamed—they laughed, "We thought food-combining was the answer to all ills!"

What had gone wrong? How was it possible that we found ourselves outside an emergency pharmacy at 2 A.M. pouring bright red deconges- tant down my six-month-old baby daughter's throat? She was a breast- fed baby! How could her nose be so blocked that she could not feed from me? Was food-combining truly the answer?

I went back to the books and after intensive research I became con- vinced that dairy products were the culprit. I decided to persist with food-combining and to see what would happen if we eliminated all dairy products from our diet. This time the change was even more dramatic. Suddenly everyone in the house began to breathe properly. Melissa, who had always slept with an open mouth (problems with her adenoids, I was told), could breathe with her mouth closed; Marie-Claire, who suf- fered from allergic rhinitis (runny nose), had a dry nose; Meredith, who had suffered from ear infections and a blocked nose, was now free of those symptoms. We were all free from the respiratory complaints that we had accepted as part of our lives. I have tested the family on numer- ous occasions since. For two or three days I have introduced a small bit of cheese, milk, or even yogurt, and the results were immediate mu- cus-related problems—ear infections, tonsillitis, post nasal drips, runny noses, blocked noses. And the best way to clear this up is not with an- tibiotics, but through a high-fruit diet, plenty of fresh vegetables, and absolutely no dairy products.

I have learned an important lesson during my years of health experi- mentation and research: *the body heals itself if you let it.*

My family has not had any health problems for twenty years now (since 1986). No ear infections. No tonsillitis. No allergies. No indigestion. No health problems of any kind! In fact, we make no medical claims due to illness on our tax return. Imagine—no antibiotics, no decongestants, no antacids, no headache tablets, no nasal sprays, in fact, no medication at all since we changed the way we ate; best of all, no wasted time sitting in doctors' waiting rooms with sick children.

How Did We Do It?

More health foods, more vitamins? No! By changing our lifestyle, by spending less time in the kitchen and more time with one another.

I must add here that I definitely do not know everything there is to know about the human body and nutrition (even after close to thirty years of researching natural health and nutrition), and I've yet to encounter anyone else who does. I only know that I'll spend the rest of my life studying this fascinating subject, and if in the process I can help anyone who has suffered the irritating symptoms of normal, modern life, then I will feel that I have achieved something worthwhile.

In the following chapters I've included practical information on how to get started on the road to perfect health the natural way, and I have included research information available both locally and abroad. Don't allow yourself to become discouraged on this road to natural health; keep looking back to see how far you have come, and you'll be motivated to keep going.

I pray that God gives you the wisdom and the perseverance as you start on the road back to your given right: Perfect Health.

CHAPTER TWO

Why Do We Become Sick and Overweight?

OVER THE YEARS as I have traveled across the world and spoken to people of different races, colors, creeds, religions, and languages, I ask a few questions and have always been given the same answers.

The first question I ask is, "How many of you are confused about your health?" Virtually everyone raises their hands. The second question is, "How many of you crave sweet foods?" Half the room raises their hands. The third question is, "How many of you crave salty foods?" The other half of the room raises their hands. The fourth and final question is, "How many of you have been on various diets and how many of you are unhappy with your health?" At which point usually everyone raises both hands.

Why Do We Get Sick in the First Place?

Most of us are continually on diets and very few of us are happy with our health—why do we become sick and overweight? What exactly are we missing?

If I look at the thousands of letters and e-mails I have received since 1991 when I wrote my first book, and if I look at the wide range of symptoms people have, I begin to realize how mainstream poor health really is.

There are those of you who suffer from bowel problems, ranging from constipation to irritable bowel syndrome and Crohn's disease, those with reproductive problems from endometriosis to polycystic ovarian syndrome, premenstrual tension and severe menopausal symptoms, infertility and sterility, no libido. Others have headaches, insomnia, depression, allergies, hay fever, arthritis, gout, mood swings, acne, eczema, high and low blood pressure and blood sugar, insulin resistance, metabolic syndrome, weight issues, appetite problems, compulsive overeating. Need I go on? I am sure you get the point and probably identify with some of the symptoms.

The situation is getting progressively worse. Just recently I was frantically contacted to help a twenty-five-year-old man who had been hospitalized for a mysterious ailment that no one could diagnose. His muscles were so weak he could not stand or drive his car. Various doctors at three separate hospitals had done every known test on him and as a last resort he contacted his brother who knows me personally.

Within three days of changing to a totally raw plant-based diet, 60 percent of the symptoms had disappeared! Within a week he was driving his car, and I just received an e-mail stating he has never felt this good in his entire life! He is also one of the people we interview in one of our Digimags. A week later I received another call, this time a seventeen-year-old with the same problem—unable to get out of bed. It seems that a generation of junk-food diets is resulting in these strange conditions. The chickens have come home to roost and the results are quite frightening. (Both these young men lived on junk-food diets.) The wonderful thing is that when we treat our bodies the way they were designed to be fed, it responds with good health—always.

The huge study undertaken by Cornell and Oxford Universities and the Chinese Academy of Preventative Health shows that diet plays a tremendous role in disease and obesity. This, the largest and most comprehensive nutritional study conducted to date, involved the diet of thousands of Chinese men and women. The researchers found that these people have high-plant, unprocessed, low-protein content in their diet as opposed to the refined, highly processed, and additive-laden diet typical of many Western countries. The study shows that the diet of the rural Chinese promotes health, whereas that of the typical Westerner promotes disease. When I mention this, many people comment that the Chinese have a different genetic makeup and they are stronger than people in the West. But when the Chinese live in the West they develop the same diseases we have (*The China Study* 234).

An article appeared in the July 6, 1963 issue of *The Lancet*, a highly reputable medical journal, showing that people in Northwest Pakistan (the Hunzas) consume the simplest possible diet of wheat, corn, potatoes, and fruit. No connection was made between their diet and their state of well-being. These people trudged up and down the rough mountain paths for anything up to fifty miles a day. Virtually no refined sugar was consumed and their remarkable physical fitness, absence of obesity, cavity-free teeth, and longevity have been cited with astonishment.

At that time it appeared researchers thought there was some miracle substance or nutrient in the glacier water they drank. It always amazes me how people look for a miracle substance or nutrient instead of looking at a whole lifestyle. Unfortunately, a Westernized diet has slowly been introduced to these people over the years, and they no longer have a clear health record (*Hunza Health Secrets*).

It is clear that diet plays a tremendous role in maintaining or destroying our health. Don't try to pretend that stress and pollution are the root cause—these never result in dental decay, obesity, or blocked arteries—diet, and diet alone, is to blame.

So what, in our diets, is causing our health problems?

- Our diet is predominantly acid-forming
- Our diet is too high in animal fats and proteins
- Our diet contains many harmful additives
- Our diet is too processed and refined

Each of these issues is dealt with separately and in detail in upcoming chapters, but all you need to know for now is that our bodies are simply not designed to handle these foods on a regular basis and that when we daily consume the standard American diet, something will go wrong; it just depends on genetic makeup as to what will go wrong and when.

In addition, we also live incorrectly—this is where stress and pollution come in:

- Too much stress
- Too little exercise
- Too little or too much sunshine
- Too little fresh air

Combining these incorrect dietary and living habits results in many health problems, including fatigue, cellulite, excess weight, cravings, binging, insomnia, dark circles under the eyes, headaches, depression, reproductive disorders, pre-menstrual tension, premature aging, and a host of more serious diseases such as autoimmune diseases, diabetes, heart disease, and cancer, to name a few. I have included such things as fatigue and cravings deliberately, as most people think that these are normal. Believe me, they are not! Perfect health is normal. A normal response to food is with a normal healthy appetite, and a glowing complexion, shining hair, and boundless energy!

Why are we so confused?

Well, because we live in the Information Age where we have access to so much information, and most of it is conflicting and confusing, especially when it comes to health issues.

Anyone can write a book these days and, believe me, most people do! Then we have the Internet, a marvelous tool for research and an equally marvelous tool for confusion. Anyone with an opinion, product, or fad to push has his or her own Web site, newsletter, and range of products to sell.

Magazines, books, journals, and newspapers are available at affordable prices on every street corner, and each one has a conflicting column or page on what good health is. Advertisements scream from the pages, telling us why a product is good, better, or best.

First, the high-carbohydrate diet is the way; then it is high carbohydrates minus the fats; then it is low carbohydrates and no fat; then high protein, no carbohydrates, no fat; then high protein, high fat; then the guru Dr. Atkins of high-protein and high-fat diets dies of heart disease and we are back to high protein, no fat, with some vegetables?!

Margarine is better than butter; then margarine is worse than butter because it is high in trans-fatty acids that cause heart disease (which they do). "Drink milk" campaigns are poured down our throats in schools and from billboards, and then milk is found to be the main cause of many diseases, including Type 1 Diabetes. To add insult to injury everyone we meet is trying to sell us the latest miracle supplement from coral to seaweed, fish oil to "natural" caffeine.

With all this information, new books, gurus, and fads, weight and obesity have increased worldwide and our health has deteriorated. Go figure!

In 1995 there were 200 million obese people in the world. By 2003 the number had increased to 300 million. Obesity in the U.S., where new diets come out weekly, is up by more than 50 percent in an eight-year period! "Obesity is spreading to parts of the world that once worried about getting enough to eat. The health risks are as enormous as our waistlines," shouted *Newsweek* on August 11, 2003.

When I first started speaking publicly about diet in the late 1980s, the incidence of cancer in most Western countries was one person out of every six or seven. Today in 2007 that has increased to one in every three to four people.

Not only is the occurrence of cancer rising and is looking to overtake heart disease as the leading cause of death in the world, but diabetes has reached epidemic proportions in the United States.

The diet industry in the U.S. is worth $35 billion. In South Africa (a country the size of Texas) one diet organization sells more than $12 million worth of products a year, and that is in a so-called third-world country where malnutrition and related diseases are still out of control and yet obesity is increasing dramatically. Half of all South Africans are overweight or obese and 22 percent of all children ages one to nine are either overweight or obese. The reason cited by the South African Medical Research Council for this problem is mainly the migration of people from rural areas, where they eat a low-protein, high plant-based natural diet, to the urban areas where their diet takes on a more affluent Western approach with more fat, more protein, and more refined sugar and processed foods.

With all these new diets, foods, and products, obesity, disease, malnutrition, and behavioral and mental problems (including depression) are more of a problem than ever before.

Large food companies are behind most of the mainstream dietary information, with dietetics at most universities being funded by these and drug (pharmaceutical) companies. This in turn filters down to our schools where we are taught the food pyramid and how eating all things in moderation will stand us in good stead. Does anyone even know what "all things" or "moderation" means? And when will these food companies and dieticians finally accept that they are part of the problem? Probably never...unless forced to, like the cigarette industry. So until then, it is up to you to find the truth and do what you know is best for your body and your health.

People are focusing on the wrong thing: energy (calories or kJ) over nutritional value, so they remove the fat, add more artificial additives and flavors, and ignore the impact on their health. If we stopped and did just one thing—focused on our health and not our weight—we would find it a lot easier to separate the truth from the myths. Amazingly, when overweight people focus on becoming healthy, the weight just drops off on its own without them weighing and measuring themselves or their food.

So, in this chapter and the next, I will give you three guidelines to sort out the myths and misconceptions from the truth and then I will include three steps to basic health. That way, you can see just how easy and how much fun it is to follow Perfect Health. You can immediately get going as you continue to read and find out how you are supposed to treat this amazing body you were given without charge, but also with no return options. The great news is that you do not have to give anything up; at this stage you will only be adding more natural foods to your existing diet.

Three Guidelines to Less Confusion

1. Remember the K.I.S.S. principle.
2. Check out the research.
3. Learn to listen to your body.

GUIDELINE 1: Remember the K.I.S.S. Principle

"Keep it simple, stupid," or if you prefer the polite version, "Keep it straight and simple."

I am reminded here of the story we all heard as children, *The Emperor's New Clothes* by Hans Christian Andersen. Remember how two con-artists approached the emperor with the latest, most expensive new fabric on the market. It was such special cloth that only really brilliant, clever people could see it (or so they said). Anyway, the day came when he had to wear these amazing clothes in a procession. The people all oohed and aahed as they too had heard that only really smart people could see these clothes, but it was up to a very simple young child to see that the emperor was in fact stark naked and said so aloud.

Well, it's a bit like that with our health. There are dozens of diets and products all claiming to be the miracle cure or answer to your problems, but they are complicated and because we assume we are stupid and don't know anything we just accept a lot of this information without questioning it.

We need to be as little children and say, "This does not make any sense!" We need to learn to trust our instincts and not be intimidated by people's credentials, how many books they have written, what scientific terminology they use, or how many television shows they have been on.

Does it make any sense that only wealthy, educated people have the right to be healthy? Of course not. But if you look at these diets they imply as much. Take the blood-group diet, for example: this diet says we are to eat according to the four main blood groups. It makes crazy claims about type-A blood group not being able to eat mangoes and type-O blood group not being able to eat avocados, two extremely nutritious foods found in abundance in third-world countries.

Imagine saying to a poor, uneducated family who just happened to live under a mango tree that they could not eat one of the most nutritious foods around simply because they have type-A blood. They would look at you as if you had lost your mind. First, they have no idea what blood group means and second, they probably have better health than the person who wrote the book on the blood-group diet! And how would any family cope if they had all four blood groups and had to prepare four different meals?! The dietary principles you follow should be affordable to all.

I suppose that living in Africa for most of my life has made me realize just how foolish these crazy programs are. Imagine going up to a poor African family whose staple food is potatoes and telling them not to eat the potatoes because the Glycemic Index (GI) or Glycemic Load (GL) is too high. They too would shake their heads and walk away in shock at this crazy person.

The blood-group diet and the GI or GL diets have helped some people, but mainly because they are told to exclude any processed foods from their diet. Anyone's health would improve if they did that, regardless of blood group or economic status.

Can you imagine telling your five-year-old son or daughter not to eat pineapple because the GI is too high? If you went with this approach, it would mean that refined white sugar is better than many fresh fruits, and fries are better than a baked potato!

But anyone of any race, color, creed, age, income group, religion, or educational level can understand that we have God-made bodies and if we put God-made food into God-made bodies it will result in God-made health. If we put man-made food into God-made bodies we end up with man-made diseases. And yes, I have tested this approach out on small children and uneducated, poor people and they all understand and it makes sense to them.

So, the next time you are confused about dietary information ask yourself, *Can a small child or a poor, uneducated person understand this and afford this?* If the answer is *no* then you should not be doing it, either.

Perfect Health is just that simple. It is about eating food that our bodies are biologically designed to eat.

Most veterinarians will tell you not to give your dog chocolate as the theobromine in the cocoa beans can kill dogs, and most of us will take more care and pay more attention to feeding our dogs and cats and servicing our motor vehicles than we do to the irreplaceable body that we are born with. You can buy a new car any time you can afford it, but there is no one in the world who can buy a new body (even if *Extreme Makeover* wants you to think you can).

Two of the richest men who ever lived, Aristotle Onassis and Howard Hughes, died prematurely (and unnecessarily) of diseases that could have been prevented by diet and lifestyle changes that would not have cost them a cent.

The wonderful thing is that health is freely available to everyone; all you have to do is use basic common sense and make better choices. The information in this book will help you do just that and the first three steps make it simple enough for anyone to follow.

As simple as these steps are, it took me ten years of battling with my health and reading just about every book I could get my hands on to reach this point. I found that many of the people I respected and who had genuine glowing health followed one basic premise, that the body will repair and heal itself if it is fed the right, natural foods.

These principles go back to the creation of man. To quote Genesis 1:29, "Then God said, 'I give you every seed-bearing plant on the face of the whole earth and every tree that has fruit with seed in it. They will be yours for food.'"

During the time of Hippocrates (460–377 B.C.), these principles were being applied. Known as the father of modern medicine, Hippocrates regarded the human body as a whole organism and he treated his patients in what we would call a holistic manner, with proper diet, fresh air, and attention to lifestyle habits and living conditions.

Then there were people such as Florence Nightingale, who insisted on fresh air, sunshine, wholesome food, and spotlessly clean accommodations for her patients, at a time when the notions of good hygiene were not widespread.

Men such as Dr. William Hay, Dr. Herbert Shelton, Dr. Henry Bieler, and Dr. Robert S. Mendelsohn are all contemporary medical doctors who became disillusioned with what modern medicine had to offer. They realized that there is no sense in treating the symptom without first seeking out the cause. In most instances, the cause was found to be incorrect eating and poor lifestyle habits. These men did extensive work and documented their findings in numerous books. In 1935 Dr. William Hay's *A New Health Era* was published. Dr. Hay was a medical practitioner who lost faith in the abilities of medicine when he became ill with a so-called incurable disease. He was spurred on to research and study how lifestyle and diet affect health. To quote from the conclusion of his book: "To live right, so as to cost us nothing in dissipated vitality, is easier than to live wrong" (*A New Health Era*). He managed to recover and live to a ripe old age.

In 1965 Dr. Bieler, a medical practitioner from Capistrano Beach, recorded the findings of his research about how diet affects health in his book *Food Is Your Best Medicine*. Similarly, Dr. Mendelsohn published his findings in the 1980s in *Confessions of a Medical Heretic*. Dr. Shelton, another medical man who practiced from the 1930s to the 1980s, is the author of many books on the subject of health, lifestyle, and diet, and he did much to capture the principles of natural health in his writings. His books include: *Superior Nutrition*; *Health for the Millions*; *Living Life to Live it Longer*; *Exercise!*; *Food Combining Made Easy*; and *Hygienic Care of Children*—all invaluable sources of information.

The interesting thing about these men and their research is that their work and findings were totally independent of one another, and yet they seemed to reach much the same conclusion. Namely, that the body is supremely intelligent and, if treated correctly and fed simply, it will always heal itself. They also discovered that by living correctly the quality of life is greatly improved.

Most recently Dr. T. Colin Campbell published his findings from the most comprehensive study of nutrition ever conducted to date in his book, *The China Study*. If you read no other book on health except *The*

China Study, your life will be forever changed. Everything in all the books I have read on natural health and all we, as a family, have done for more than twenty years is confirmed in this book.

The research took twenty years, two top universities (Cornell and Oxford University), and thousands of people in China through the Chinese Academy of Preventative Medicine (no wonder the Chinese are shooting way ahead in the world economy—they have an academy that focuses on preventing disease, not just attempting to find cures for sick people) and in the end they found what thousands have been doing and saying since the beginning of time.

Feed and look after your body the way it was designed to be fed and looked after and you will be healthy. It's that simple.

GUIDELINE 2: Check Out the Research

The second thing to look at when trying to find the truth is: who paid for the research? Often people, books, and magazines make claims about research but they seldom tell you where their research came from and who paid for it. I remember being on national television in South Africa with a nutritional guru from the U.K. He was flown out and sponsored by a large vitamin-producing company and on-air he made some wild claims about how research shows that supplements can restore your health. At which point I interrupted him and asked why more than 5,000 studies indicate that supplements are of no value to our health as we can only use 4–10 percent of the nutrients in supplements and, in fact, they can actually damage our health. These studies clearly indicated that people who ate more unprocessed foods and more fruits and vegetables benefited from improved health. I also asked him who paid for the research. He never answered (I since found out it was the supplement companies he represented), but he did say that most people will not eat fruits and vegetables, and that 4–10 percent was better than nothing!

Look at how many supplements and health-related products are out there, yet our health is getting worse, and we continue to be impressed when companies produce an article showing research that backs their products. Ninety to 96 percent of your hard-earned money is being urinated into the toilet and flushed away when you take vitamin supplements!

For years, the dairy industry has been telling us that milk, milk products, yogurt, and cheese will prevent osteoporosis (brittle bone disease), yet the countries that consume the most milk and milk products have the most osteoporosis cases and the countries that consume the least dairy have the least brittle bone disease.

One of the most powerful things about the Internet is that it makes it so easy to check out research. Genuine research will indicate who funded it and usually you have to pay to download the research in full.

Genuine research has nothing to gain from telling you the information; no one is getting rich in the process.

I do strongly suggest that you get a copy of *The China Study*. It really is the definitive book on nutritional research. Once you have read *The China Study*, chances are you will never be confused again, and, if you do get confused by some slick sales pitch, read it again and again until it really sinks in. You simply cannot argue with this work and those that try to are the ones who have never read it in the first place and/or are trying to protect their incomes. The book is available from the publisher at www.benbellabooks.com.

I have found all other independent research ties in and confirms this huge study. The minute it does not, I check out the funding and find it is backed by someone with an economic motive.

And, whereas *The China Study* will tell you why you should change your diet and lifestyle, *Perfect Health* will tell you why and *how* to change your diet and lifestyle.

RECAP

- Keep it simple—health should be accessible to all, and remember *The Emperor's New Clothes*
- Look at independent research based on real people

CHAPTER THREE

Listening to Your Body

YOUR BODY is incredibly intelligent. Learn to listen to it. This leads me to the third guideline in your search for truth when it comes to your health.

GUIDELINE 3: Learn to Listen to Your Body

Our bodies have natural recurring cycles. We need to sleep every twenty-four hours, although the amount of sleep needed differs from person to person. We also need to eat and drink at regular intervals, and our bowels need to be emptied at least every twenty-four hours (in healthy individuals this is usually first thing in the morning). Women have a monthly cycle in which they ovulate approximately every twenty-eight days.

Scientists now accept that all living organisms have natural cycles. These are sometimes referred to as *circadian rhythms*. In learning to listen to our bodies, we need to tune into our natural body cycles. A good way to start is by understanding what happens when we sleep. While we are asleep, our bodies automatically step up their repair and cleansing operation. To assist the body in this we need to feed it properly. When, for example, we eat a very heavy evening meal that is also poorly combined, the body is using most of its energy to sort out the mess in the stomach. The result is that the repair, cleansing, and rebuilding that should take place have been neglected.

We then wake up after eight hours of sleep feeling totally exhausted.

The most obvious benefit that you will enjoy after your change to the Perfect Health principles is that you'll wake up feeling alive and well-rested. Your food will have been digested before you even fall asleep and your body can carry out its normal rhythmical chores while you sleep, which means that you will wake up full of vigor. When you get up in the morning, your body has to eliminate the resultant debris from its repairing and cleansing work. This will be done through the bladder, bowels, and other body orifices such as the nose or mouth. Have you ever noticed how a mucus problem is usually worse in the morning and tends to dry up toward lunch-time? This is because your body steps up its elimination first thing in the morning to get rid of the accumulated waste products of the night. This is one of the normal healthy cycles of your body. To facilitate this function, you need to feed the body something that is easy to digest and that won't direct energy away from its cleansing efforts. One of the best foods for this would be fresh fruit.

The human body is incredibly intelligent and wise, and by respecting that intelligence, the quality of life improves.

Take something as simple as thirst.

When your cells (everything ultimately happens at a cellular level) have not received enough water with the last intake of food, or if the intake contained too much salt or other condiments (your body needs more water to dilute the toxic effect that the condiments or salt would have on the cells), they set about obtaining the water that they need to function. The cells send a message to the brain, the brain interprets the message, and your throat becomes dry. You then realize that you are thirsty and you drink something. The cells have obtained their water and can go about their business once more. Now all that took place without your being aware of it! Well, other than your reaching for that glass of water.

Then, of course, there is that miracle of conception and growth in the uterus. What tells the fertilized egg to divide and multiply? What tells it to develop some cells that will form a heart and others that will form the lungs? What tells it to form certain organs of the body before others? It can only be the God-created, innate intelligence of the body. Yet we treat our bodies badly; we become ill and then expect something as inanimate as an antibiotic to have more intelligence than this wondrous and complex organism.

Think of the sun, for example. Our bodies need about twenty minutes of sunshine a day. But what do we do? We lie in the sun and after twenty minutes we begin to feel hot and uncomfortable. Do we get out of the sun? No! We jump into the sea or a swimming pool to cool down so that we can force our bodies to take more sunshine than they need. The result? Burning, sunstroke, and even skin cancer! We then say that the sun is dangerous and go to great lengths to stay out of it and our health suffers in the long term. We constantly demonstrate our lack of respect for our body's intelligence.

As new-born babies we know instinctively how to listen to our bodies and even as young children we are still aware of its messages. But as we grow older, we forget how to listen, and eventually become deaf to them. A small child or baby will not want to eat when he or she is not well. The body is trying to focus all its energy on correcting the problem at hand and does not want any food in the stomach as digestion requires a great deal of energy. The body, in the meantime, always makes sure that it stores reserves for times like these. So what do we clever adults do? "The child won't eat," we say. "The child will die if he doesn't eat." So we proceed to tempt the child with all kinds of treats, non-foods that in the long run pervert the child's taste buds and do more damage than if he had not eaten at all. Remember being fed Jell-o and ice cream when you weren't well as a child? Remember being coaxed to eat so that you could get well sooner? Well, you didn't get well sooner. All that happened was you were taught not to listen to your body.

I am not trying to blame our parents for all our bad eating habits (although when I look around and see how parents today just allow a three-year-old to dictate his or her choice of food, maybe I should!), but I am merely trying to show how we learned not to listen to our bodies.

So here we are, years later, and we crave sweet and savory foods on a daily basis. Do we stop for a minute and ask exactly what it is that our body needs? No. Of course not. We reach for a chocolate bar or a packet of potato chips or fries and carry on thinking we must be suffering from a chocolate or potato-chip deficiency.

The most common reason we crave sweets is that our brains and central nervous systems cannot work without glucose, our hearts cannot pump without glucose, our lungs cannot breathe without glucose, and each cell requires glucose just to function. If all you did was sit in a chair and breathe you would need glucose (but obviously at a lower rate than someone who jogs an hour a day). The way your cells tell you they need glucose is by sending a message to the brain and the brain interprets the signal by sending a message to the taste buds to crave sweet things.

The normal response to sugar cravings is to reach for a candy bar, chocolate, maybe tea or coffee with two spoons of sugar, a chocolate-chip cookie, a donut, a can of soda, or even an alcoholic beverage.

The response from the body is almost immediate: your blood sugar shoots up to dangerous levels, and your body reacts by producing loads of insulin to bring it back down. As your blood sugar rises you feel energized and alive, but as it starts to come back down you feel lethargic, flat, tired, and even depressed as it reaches its low point, at which you crave sweets again and the whole cycle starts over.

"So what's the problem?" you may ask. "I am listening to my body, aren't I?" Yes, you are, but you are interpreting the signals incorrectly.

First, when your blood sugar is upset like this, three systems are also upset: the brain and central nervous system, the immune system, and the endocrine system.

This could result in moodiness, mood swings, depression, poor concentration, feeling "spaced out," and generally having a brain that does not work as efficiently as it was designed to. When the immune system is upset you could come down with anything from a sore throat to serious colds, flu, or even autoimmune diseases, and when the endocrine system is upset it upsets all the hormones and these (over two dozen chemical messengers) control almost every function of the body. Anything could go wrong at this point, from high or low blood pressure and/or blood sugar, to allergies, hay fever, constipation, tiredness, excess weight, slow metabolism, low body weight, sped-up metabolism, poor muscle tone, poor sleep, and liver, lung, heart, skin, and kidney problems.

I can just hear you say, "Come off it, not from one lousy chocolate bar?" No, not from one chocolate bar, but if you add up all the foods and drinks we consume in a year, the average American consumes at least 130–150 pounds of sugar per annum. That is 130–150 pounds of a substance your amazing body was never designed to cope with. It is a miracle that our bodies last as long as they do.

OK, I did say you would not have to give anything up so how are you going to deal with this, and where are you going to find the right glucose?

Well, the best way to find out what your body really needs (apart from what your taste buds seem to be saying) is to place yourself back in the Garden of Eden, back to the beginning of time, when there were no shops, no fast-food outlets, no restaurants, just food growing on trees. In that environment, if you were craving something sweet, what would you eat?

Easy: maybe some fresh dates, a few bananas, grapes, apples—whatever fruit you could find. Well, the amazing thing about fruit is it is perfectly designed for your body and will not upset your blood sugar the way refined sucrose (the sugar in soda, cakes, donuts, candy, etc.) does.

The Most Perfect Food?

In most warm countries such as South Africa, Australia, and many parts of the U.S., where we have an abundance of fruit available all year round at very reasonable prices, it is surprising that so little fruit is actually consumed. Of the thousands of people that I have had the opportunity to consult with, either privately or in a seminar environment, very few ate more than one piece of fruit a day and many ate virtually none at all on a regular basis.

But fruit is in fact the most perfect food, designed specifically with man in mind. Now, many of you might throw up your hands in protest saying, "But it is so acidic and I always suffer from digestive problems when I eat fruit." Let's straighten out the misconceptions right now. Raw fruit leaves an alkaline residue in your bloodstream once digested, even the acid-tasting fruit, such as oranges, pineapples, and tangerines. Essie Honiball, who had lived on fruit and nuts for fourteen years and then submitted herself to a series of extensive tests by Professor B. J. Meyer (at the time, chairman of the physiology department at the University of Pretoria), was found to have alkaline urine. If fruit is indeed acid-forming, this result would not have been possible.

No raw, uncooked fruit, not even oranges, causes acid in the bloodstream. Some fruit might be acidic before it enters the body, and might digest in a more acidic environment than other fruits, but it is never acid-forming in the body or bloodstream unless it is eaten in a wrong combination with other foods. The reason for this is simple—fruit eaten on its own, on an empty stomach, digests in less time than other foods and leaves an alkaline residue in the bloodstream. This means it leaves more alkaline minerals (such as calcium, magnesium, potassium) in the bloodstream once it has been digested than acidic minerals (such as sulfur and phosphorus). The exception is people who are prone to rheumatoid arthritis, who appear to have an inability to break down the natural fruit acids in the digestive tract, which then get absorbed into the bloodstream and aggravate (not cause) the condition. Usually when the rest of the diet has been improved this is no longer the case.

Let's take, for example, the standard way of drinking orange juice. Usually, it accompanies something like toast or a sandwich or a bagel. Now orange juice (of the freshly squeezed variety) takes about fifteen minutes to one hour to digest and move out of the stomach. Toast or bread needs approximately two to four hours to move out of the stomach. Imagine what happens next. The juice is mixed up with the bread, through the normal action of the stomach. The orange juice is trapped in the stomach for longer than it should be because of the bread, and the natural sugar in the juice starts to ferment. The acidic value of the orange juice, in turn, inhibits the digesting ability of the starch-digesting enzyme, ptyalin, and so the partially digested starch in the bread starts to ferment. The result—indigestion!

And what gets blamed? The orange juice!

Fruit is so easy to digest because it is what we refer to as a partially digested food, meaning that the nutrients in the fruit are in their simplest form. The sugar in fruit is a simple sugar, or monosaccharide. It cannot be broken down any further. Thus, it is ready to be absorbed and assimilated directly by the body.

By making one meal a day a fruit meal, you'll find that you no longer crave sweets, because you will get enough glucose in your diet. Glucose is one of the most essential nutrients, but it must be taken in an unrefined state—as in fruit. This is your first Perfect Health step.

The protein (and, yes, there is some protein in all fruit) is in its broken-down form (amino acids) and the minerals and vitamins are in the most usable form. This is referred to by some as an organic state, meaning that these vital nutrients are bonded to a carbon molecule. This bonding is made possible by photosynthesis (the effect that natural light and sun have on plants) and cannot be duplicated in a laboratory (one of the many reasons I am not keen on vitamin and mineral supplementation). In this bonded form the nutrients are 100 percent usable. In supplements, vitamins and minerals are not bonded to a carbon molecule and, as such, are in an "inorganic" form and therefore only 4–10 percent usable. This will result in 90–96 percent of your hard-earned money ending up in the sewage system as your kidneys and stomach have to work very hard to eliminate these unbonded nutrients in your urine. The safest supplement to take is considered to be vitamin C and taking it can result in gout, arthritis, kidney stones, stomach ulcers, anemia, and osteoporosis. Therefore fruit, not expensive supplements, is one of the best ways to get natural nutrients into your body. If you feel you need more than that, then fresh vegetable and fruit juices would make far more sense.

I used to suffer from severe low blood sugar levels, or hypoglycemia, with dizzy spells and mood swings ranging to severe depression. When I included plenty of fresh fruit in my diet, this became a thing of the past. I have since seen that this is the case in many other people with whom I have consulted. Imagine no therapy or drugs; just a diet that includes plenty of fresh fruit. This brings to mind one particular case where a young woman was institutionalized for mental observation due to extremely severe depression. After various treatments it was finally discovered that her blood sugar level was quite erratic. By changing her diet to include more fruits and vegetables, and by removing refined sugar, this condition was entirely corrected. I have found that fresh fruit has a stabilizing effect on blood sugar because it contains water-soluble fibers, which slow down the rate at which fruit sugar (known as fructose, which has a more stable effect on blood sugar than refined sucrose) is absorbed. On top of this, fruit contains such a wide variety of nutrients that work together in the body to balance blood sugar. Many diabetics, and those with insulin resistance and hypoglycemia, have expressed concern over including fresh fruit in their diet; I have found that it is then best to eat acid and/or sub-acid fruit (see the food-combining chart on page 266) during the fruit meal with a quarter to half a cup of raw nuts or seeds. The nuts and seeds help slow down the absorption of the fruit sugar even more because the essential fats and protein in the nuts have a very stabilizing effect on blood sugar. If you still have a problem, eat small portions of fruit regularly throughout the day and thirty minutes before other meals rather than one large, fruit meal. In time you will find that you can handle fruit the way you were designed to.

A small percentage of people have mentioned that they actually have an allergic reaction to certain fruits such as strawberries and, sadly, mangoes (one of my favorite fruits). Although there seems to be little research on this problem, one reason I can find is that possibly, as a result of pesticide residues, some people have developed an allergic reaction to these fruits. This is a good enough reason to try and eat only organic produce if you can find it, and fortunately, most food stores these days have a good variety of organic produce.

Another reason, according to Professor Holgate, professor of clinical immunopharmacology at the University of Southampton, is that there have been changes in the immune system and in the natural bacteria in the gut. The environment in our bodies is too clean from sterilizing everything around us, and as a result, children's immune systems do not get boosted from natural bacteria. Research has shown that children who live on farms have a third fewer allergies than urban children. Contemporary home furnishings also harbor dust mites, a very common cause of allergies. So it seems the best way to live in order to avoid allergies is not to be obsessed with killing all germs. I have found that in time this allergic response to fruit can disappear, but only through a commitment to a natural lifestyle and within a few years you should be able to eat all fruits.

Fruit is truly a complete food. Vitamins and minerals (and that includes calcium and iron in every single fruit) are in a form that is ready to be absorbed and assimilated. The fats in fruit (oh yes, there is fat in every single fruit [see charts on composition of fruit at the back of the book]) are in the form of fatty acids that are ready to be absorbed and assimilated. The protein in fruit (and surprise, surprise, there is protein in every fruit [see tables]) is already in its simplest form—that of amino acids—and is ready to be absorbed and assimilated. Now you can begin to understand why fruit requires so little energy for digestion, and why it is the best food to eat when your body is trying to cleanse or detoxify itself. By eating easily digestible fruit, your body has a lot more energy available to do its cleaning and restoring.

Not only is fruit the easiest food to digest, but it is the only food that in its natural state is appealing to all our senses. Fruit looks good. Fruit tastes good. Fruit smells good. Fruit naturally feels good. In fact, you can live on a variety of fruit (including nuts, seeds, and avocado—all technically fruit) and live in perfect health.

My family has lived on a diet that contains at least three to five daily fruit portions and even more when we do a detox program (depending on the weather, the fruit, and our appetites) since 1985. The change in our health and energy levels has been phenomenal, to say the least. My own mother has followed this program for nearly as long now and has become a different person. She used to suffer continually from sinusitis, bronchitis, bladder infections, exhaustion, and a cranky disposition, and she has now become a person who is always positive and in the best of health. In fact, friends and acquaintances who have not seen her for many years have asked her, "Angelique, who did your face-lift?"

We have now seen thousands of people and their families all over the world benefit from a high intake of fresh fruit. The natural antioxidants, vitamins, and minerals help the body do repair work very efficiently and this is what helps slow down the aging process as well as keep you healthy.

It is important to remember that fruit does not do anything to your body; rather your body uses the fruit that you have eaten. Fruit causes very little strain on the body as it contains no toxic or poisonous elements such as those found in virtually every other food.

For example, certain vegetables such as spinach contain oxalic acid, which prevents the absorption of iron. Harmful substances such as mustard oil, an irritant to the digestive track, and allicin, a natural antibiotic, are usually found together in garlic or onions. Simply because allicin is a natural antibiotic does not make it any better than a pharmaceutically prepared one. An antibiotic is a destructive substance ("anti" means "against" and "biotic" means "life"). It destroys both harmful and friendly bacteria and can disturb the natural intestinal flora or bacteria. Once the balance has been destroyed in the digestive tract, candida albicans, a natural yeast that occurs in our digestive tracts, multiplies uncontrollably, causing health problems. Pernicious anemia is another likely problem as vitamin B12 is manufactured in the human body in the small intestine by the natural bacteria or flora that are so easily destroyed by antibiotics.

According to J. I. Rodale in his book, *The Complete Book of Food and Nutrition*, Dr. Kalser of the University of Illinois conducted experiments on himself, medical students, and dogs, in which the effect of onion consumption resulted in anemia. It was found that the red blood cell and hemoglobin count were starkly reduced with an increased intake of onion.

It has been found that by cooking onion and garlic much of the effect of these properties is reduced. This is one of the reasons why a cooked onion is so much sweeter than a raw one. The stronger the bite of onion or garlic, the more concentrated the mustard oil and allicin. Mustard oil is also metabolized as thiocyanate in the body, which has been found to suppress the production of the hormone thyroxin from the thyroid gland. This, in turn, can slow down the metabolism of the body and result in weight problems and other disorders such as constipation, fuzzy head, and dry skin.

Many grains contain gluten and phytic acid. A great number of people have been found to have intolerance to gluten, which results in various digestive problems, from distension to diarrhea. Gluten has now been found to upset the delicate balance of the hormonal system and immune system, resulting in autoimmune diseases such as diabetes, lupus, and multiple sclerosis, as well as reproductive problems. Phytic acid, which prevents the absorption of calcium, and gluten are found in all wheat products such as bread, cookies, and cakes.

All animal products contain saturated fats and cholesterol and high levels of a fatty acid known as arachidonic acid, known to encourage inflammatory conditions such as gout and arthritis and encourage blood clotting, which contributes to heart disease. All these substances place a strain on the body and its functions. Fruit contains none of these.

For the skeptics, hear what Professor B. J. Meyer has to say on the subject in his book *Fruit for Thought:* "By consuming adequate quantities of fruit, a subject can supply his total protein requirements...it is clear that a fruitarian diet can supply the recommended calcium allowances...[and that] a balanced fruit diet will supply the recommended daily iron allowances" (48–50). Professor Meyer ends by saying that "Considering all the pros and cons, it is my firm conviction that from a health point of view, a fruit diet, including nuts and unrefined cereals, has much to be recommended" (50).

Okay! Don't panic, you don't have to become a fruitarian to attain a better level of health. You don't even have to become a vegetarian. You can choose what changes you want to make and how soon you want to make them. Remember, it's your body! I am just trying to illustrate how essential fresh fruit is to a healthy diet.

In brief:

- Fruit contains all the nutrients we need
- Fruit allows the body to cleanse and repair itself
- Fruit in its natural state is appealing to all our senses
- All fruit leaves an alkaline residue or end product in the body
- Fruit regulates your blood sugar

If you follow Step 1 of Perfect Health you will find yourself satisfying the body's need for glucose and supplying yourself with ample vitamins, minerals, and antioxidants so that you will save yourself the cost of expensive, useless supplements, while at the same time benefiting your health.

STEP 1: Eat One Fruit Meal a Day

Try to eat one meal every day that comprises of only fresh fruit. This can be as much as you like but not less than two pieces. There is no limit and no measuring; simply eat as much as you like until you feel satisfied. If you feel fruit is not enough and have blood sugar problems, eat mainly acid and sub-acid fruit and include a quarter to half a cup of raw unsalted nuts (almonds, cashews, pecans, Brazil nuts), or seeds such as sunflower and pumpkin seeds.

This meal can be eaten at any time of the day, but I have found that most people prefer eating their fruit meal in the morning.

STEP 2: Snack on Raw Fruit or Vegetables Before You Eat Refined Sugar or Heated Fats

Each time you crave something sweet, first eat one to two pieces of fresh fruit or up to half a cup of preservative-free dried fruit such as raisins or dates.

So what about those salty foods you crave?

I have found the most common reason we crave savory foods is a lack of essential fats in out diets. Take a look at the foods you reach for when craving these foods: fries, potato chips, hamburgers, cheese, pizza, toasted sandwiches, etc.—all high in fats.

Your endocrine system (remember, this is the system that controls all those hormones that control almost every function in your body such as blood pressure, blood sugar, weight, metabolism, sleep, and liver, kidney, skin, heart, and lung function) cannot function without essential fatty acids.

Now, much has been made about these fatty acids, known as Omega 3 and Omega 6, and in chapter eight I will clear up some of the confusion surrounding them, but for now all you need to know is that basically nothing will work efficiently in your body if you lack them.

These fatty acids are what your cells are telling your brain you need, and again our poor taste buds scream out for fries and cheese and of course, we quite comfortably satisfy them.

Consider what you would eat in the Garden of Eden that grows on trees or out of the ground that is naturally high in fats. Nuts, avocado, seeds, sweet corn on the cob, and oils cold-pressed from the plant source. I can just hear you screaming "High fat! We cannot eat those!" Just relax. Your body will not work properly without them and in chapter eight I will give you quantities and explain exactly why you need them. What you need to remember is every time you crave salty foods, first eat some natural plant foods containing fats. This is the second part of Step 2.

You can eat candy or fries, if you still feel like it. In time, as you learn to listen to your body, your taste buds will change and as your cells begin to receive the nutrients they need, they will stop sending frantic messages to your brain, and amazingly, you will stop being controlled by food!

Fruit is certainly not the only plant food you should be eating. Vegetables and grains have their place, too. Fruit is very high in vitamins and antioxidants and is a valuable source of carbohydrates in a broken-down and very usable form, and vegetables are a wonderful source of many minerals and antioxidants. Vegetables are also alkaline in our bloodstream and what we know from most independent research is that we need to be following a 75–80 percent alkaline-forming diet. Research from Britain shows that the higher the alkaline environment in the brain, the higher the IQ. And the way to create a higher alkaline environment in the body is to eat more alkaline-forming foods.

Alkaline-forming foods are all fruit and vegetables, millet (a grain that grows naturally in Africa with very little water), and almonds. The rest of our foods are acid-forming in varying degrees. This does not mean you cannot eat acid-forming foods, just that they should not form more than 25 percent of your daily intake. The first three steps will help you do this. It is also known that the more balanced the acid/alkaline ratio, the less chance you have of developing degenerative diseases such as cancer. The higher the alkaline in your diet, the easier it is to convert fuel (food) into energy, which will help you attain the right weight. *The China Study* clearly showed how even though the rural Chinese ate more in energy value than the average U.S. diet provided, there were considerably fewer people carrying extra weight. The Chinese eat more fruit and vegetables than the average American.

STEP 3: Start All Cooked Meals with Raw Vegetables

Start all cooked meals (especially lunch and supper) with a medium plate of raw, uncooked vegetables. This can be a salad or strips of raw vegetables with a dip, a glass of carrot or fresh tomato juice, or a cucumber for that matter. (For ideas, see the recipe section or our Web site, www.mary-anns.com.) British nutritionist and immunologist Jennifer Meek found that starting your cooked meals with raw vegetables prevented destruction of white blood cells, which is important in maintaining a healthy immune system and one of the steps we always follow regardless of where we are. Including this third step in your program will give you the 75 percent alkaline-forming diet that will help you be smarter, healthier, and slimmer.

RECAP

- Listen to your body and eat fresh fruit before you eat anything else that's sweet
- Eat foods containing natural fats before you eat foods containing animal or processed fats
- Follow the first three steps to make sure you have a high alkaline-forming diet

CHAPTER FOUR

The Ins and Outs of Digestion

*"You can't ignore the importance of good digestion;
the joy of life depends on a sound stomach."*

—DR. JOSEPH CONRAD

THE QUESTIONS I get asked most often (and usually in private after I have done a talk) are about constipation, indigestion, bloating, and flatulence. That fact that the second most commonly bought over-the-counter medication (after painkillers) is antacid and digestive medication shows how prevalent the issue of digestion is.

Many people have more working knowledge of their car engine than their digestive tract, so I think a basic lesson in digestion in this chapter will help you take control of your digestive tract and get rid of those irritating and sometimes debilitating digestive problems.

I remember how Mark and I used to suffer from indigestion after virtually every meal. It wasn't that we ate rich meals, it just seemed to be par for the course. Antacid preparations were always in the house, and in fact, they were a permanent fixture on my shopping list. Whether we went to a barbecue, ate roasted chicken and potatoes at home, or had a simple supper of toasted sandwiches or a cheese omelet, we always suffered from indigestion.

Another thing we suffered from was continual exhaustion. We slept our weekends away. Saturdays we slept (usually in front of the television) and Sundays we collapsed on the bed after lunch for a few hours. Mark used to say that he felt as if he were sleeping his life away.

The reason I mention these symptoms is that many people suffer from them, and don't realize that this is far from normal. Normal is having boundless energy and never suffering from indigestion, flatulence, or constipation. Normal is having a digestive system of which you are not even aware. In other words, normal is having no reflux, no ulcers, no spastic colons, or any other digestive-related problem. Over years of counseling and speaking to people about their diets, everyone who has had any digestive problem has improved by following the Perfect Health principles.

Then there were my so-called "allergy" problems. No amount of medication did anything to relieve my painful symptoms. I had suffered from severe dermatitis or eczema on the palms of my hands for more than four years, and my nose had been streaming for more than a year. Nothing made any difference and yet I had tried every medical and non-medical avenue open to me: cortisone creams, nasal sprays, homeopathic remedies, and vitamin supplements. I had no idea that these problems were related to my digestive tract.

It was only when we started combining our food correctly after reading the book *Food Combining for Health* that I experienced immediate relief. My nose stopped running instantly and my hands took about four days to stop itching and clear up. With our new, properly combined eating regime, indigestion became a thing of the past and our energy levels soared. Two months later we were so well we had almost forgotten what we had felt like before and went back to our old way of eating. The result—instant indigestion, a streaming nose, and the little tell-tale blisters appeared between my fingers, plus the exhaustion had returned. We certainly did not need any more proof that food-combining worked. But as always, that was not enough for me. I wanted to know how and why it worked. How could eating the same foods but at different times affect our energy and well-being?

I started my research by reading as many books on the subject of digestion as I could get my hands on—going so far as to dig into the medical library archives at the local university. I read books such as *The Work of the Digestive System* by Professor Ivan Pavlov and Charles Griffin (1910). And I was fascinated by the experiments performed on Alexis St. Martin by Dr. William Beaumont from 1825 to 1832. In these experiments Dr. Beaumont set out to prove that the stomach did contain a digestive enzyme. He did this by suspending different types of foods on silk threads into the stomach of St. Martin, who had a hole in his stomach caused by a gunshot wound that had not closed up. He would also record any observations made by looking through the hole into the stomach after a meal was consumed. Dr. Beaumont recorded the time it took for each meal to digest and from his observations over a few years, it was apparent that the more simple the meal, the easier it was to digest. For example, in one experiment only rice was eaten and this was out of the stomach in one hour. Whereas when potatoes and meat were eaten together, it could take anywhere from three to six and a half hours to digest. Although these experiments had little to do with food-combining (Dr. Beaumont had set out to prove that the stomach contains or secretes a digestive enzyme), they did prove that meals consisting of only one type of food took far less time and were more comfortable to digest than a meal that consisted of carbohydrates and proteins combined. The incorrect conclusion that he drew (as do many people on carbohydrate-free diets) is that there was no enzyme in the body that digested starches and therefore starches should be avoided.

Then there were the more detailed books, such as *A New Health Era* by Dr. William Hay and *Food Combining Made Easy* by Dr. Herbert Shelton. These two books explore the physiology of digestion—how your digestive system actually works. From my reading, I reached the inescapable conclusion that if you want complete health, it is essential that you combine your food properly and eat natural unprocessed foods.

Still curious about the subject, I then studied the process of digestion in Arthur Guyton's *Textbook of Medical Physiology* to make sure that everything else was accurate, and found that it was. I am amazed that so few people studying digestion don't realize that, from a chemical standpoint only, it is almost impossible to have an efficient digestive process if you eat starches and proteins at the same time. I realized the reason so few people understand this is because they are studying diseases and how to treat them with medication rather than looking for the cause of their discomfort.

But the most convincing evidence of all, as far as food-combining is concerned, is my own state of well-being, as well as the well-being of the thousands of people I have counseled or who have written to me with digestive-related ailments. To date, every person who has changed to correctly combining their food has been helped. From babies to elderly men and women, all have experienced a dramatic improvement in digestive function. To quote Dr. Hay, "Facts have always discounted theory, and always will; so get the facts for yourself and let others be satisfied with unproved theory."

So what is food-combining, or "The Great Apartheid Diet" as Professor Harry Seftel of Johannesburg's Wits Medical School calls it? Very simply, it is not eating a concentrated starch with a concentrated protein at the same meal.

STEP 4: Food-Combining

Keep your meals as simple as possible by eating only one concentrated food at each meal.

Concentrated foods are foods that make you feel full, such as starches and proteins. I will elaborate further on.

If it is as easy as that, the skeptics say, if we were not meant to mix starch and protein together, then why do these two occur naturally in all foods? Yes, they do occur naturally in all foods, but they are not found in an equally concentrated form in all foods.

The second argument favored by the skeptics is that early man could not have combined his food correctly. My answer is that early man ate simply and would not have mixed his foods. We know from research that without refrigeration, early man ate whatever food was most readily available. If he killed an animal to eat, he would have had to consume as much as possible in a relatively short period before the carcass went bad. In the absence of a fresh kill, he would quite easily have made a complete meal of the berries, fruit, roots, or tubers that he found in abundance. It is unlikely that these two sorts of meals would ever have been eaten at the same time as the food group theory had yet to be created.

What about the Food Pyramid?

If you look at how the process of mixing the food groups came about, we find that it is mainly due to a marketing plan put together after World War II, when the economy, including agriculture, needed a kick start.

What they taught in schools and colleges around the world was that to get all the nutrients you need for good health, you must mix the (then) three food groups. These were also known as the main agricultural groups, namely grain, fruits and vegetables, and animals. Grains and starches are for energy, fruits and vegetables are for vitamins and minerals, and proteins from animals are for building strength. This had very little to do with actual science and everything to do with the economy.

Within a few years the dairy industry became more powerful and wanted their own food group and a few years later so did the fat industry. Did our health improve? Absolutely not. In fact, since WWII heart disease, cancer, diabetes, obesity, autoimmune diseases, and digestive diseases increased.

As research started to show how our health had deteriorated and that we needed to be eating simpler with less protein and less processed fats, the food industry attempted to change things by introducing the food pyramid. Here there is anything from five to eleven food groups just to make sure everyone receives a share of the market. Has it helped? Absolutely not! But if you feel the need to follow a pyramid when it comes to choosing food, the University of California's food pyramid is probably the best; this is the one with fresh fruits and vegetables at the base. The one with grains at the base appears to be put together by the breakfast cereal industry. In the last year we have seen the introduction of twelve food pyramids with rainbow-colored, vertical stripes, just to confuse us further. You'd be better off ignoring all the pyramids, following the guidelines in this book, and listening to your body!

Digestion of Starches/Proteins

What is now meant by a concentrated starch is usually a food with 20 percent or more carbohydrate content. Potatoes, rice, bread, noodles, corn on the cob, and all grains such as wheat, rye, oats, etc., would fall into this category. (See food-combining chart on page 265.) These foods need to be chewed well so that the enzyme ptyalin (also known as salivary amylase), which is secreted in the saliva, can start acting on the starch. The ultimate aim is to break these starches down into simple sugars, which is the only way they can be absorbed into the bloodstream. Very simply, starch moves into the stomach, where it is churned up while the ptyalin continues to act on it. (No additional enzyme that digests starches is secreted in the stomach.) This mixture, called chyme, then passes into the small intestine where further digestion takes places with the aid of amylase or starch-splitting enzymes. The simple sugars that result from this breaking-down process are then absorbed into the bloodstream and used by the body.

Concentrated proteins are those foods that contain 15 percent or more complete protein, such as meat, chicken, fish, eggs, and some cheeses; in fact, all animal products other than the fats such as butter and cream are protein. Most nuts and seeds also fall into this category. (Refer to chart at the back of the book.) These foods digest in a somewhat different way compared with that of the concentrated starches. They are not acted on by the ptyalin but merely broken down mechanically by the teeth. The chewed protein then passes into the stomach, where hydrochloric acid is stimulated in direct proportion to the amount of protein present. Pepsin, the protein-digesting enzyme, is activated by this hydrochloric acid. The pepsin then proceeds with the action of breaking the protein down into amino acids. Further digestion takes place in the small intestine to complete the process. The body can only absorb the protein once it is in this broken-down form.

If you were looking at a line graph representing the pH balance at the time of digestion, you would find that protein digests easier, faster, and more efficiently in a more acidic environment than starch. Protein prefers a pH level from three down, whereas starch prefers a pH level of four or higher. When you combine the two together, the hydrochloric acid has a neutralizing effect on the more alkaline ptyalin, and in turn, this suspends or stops the digestion of the starch before completion. The partially digested starches then begin to ferment, thus causing the protein to putrefy. What results from this fermenting mess is alcohol, acetic acid (stronger than vinegar), and ammonia. These substances are all poisonous to the body and end up in the bloodstream with partially digested protein, contributing to a condition known as *leaky gut syndrome*. In my case, and thousands of other people, this condition results in various allergies. Gas, wind, and flatulence are also a result, as is acid indigestion or heartburn. These conditions are ideal for the hiatus hernias (also known as reflux) and spastic colons to start acting up. People with Irritable Bowel Syndrome (IBS), diverticulitis, Crohn's disease, and ulcerative colitis have all benefited from this basic principle.

As far back as 1888 Dr. James Salisbury, in his research documented in *The Relation of Alimentation and Disease*, found that starches ferment readily in the stomach, resulting in acetic acid. This in turn leads to a variety of symptoms and conditions including headaches, throat congestion, mucus expectoration (this is where my sneezing and runny nose fit in), pains in the heart, sour perspiration, alternate fever, rapid pulse, and chills (I've found that menopausal women who suffer from hot flashes are often cured when they combine properly). Dr. Salisbury even found that vinegar could, through a chain of events, cause tuberculosis. He also found that vinegar tends to leak phosphorus from the body and stimulates the thyroid gland. As phosphorus is depleted, so in turn is the function of the adrenal system. (The vinegar formed in the stomach through bad combining is no different from any other vinegar, except it is stronger. It is a by-product of fermentation. Even so-called healthy vinegars, such as apple-cider vinegar and balsamic vinegar, are fermented products and could cause the above symptoms. Fresh lemon juice is preferable if you want a tang to your food.)

As a result of the suspension of the digestive process caused by poor combining, food is not broken down completely and the maximum amount of nutrients cannot be absorbed. This results in various deficiencies. Many people with so-called iron deficiencies have had perfectly normal iron levels after only a few weeks of correct food-combining.

It can also double the time it takes to digest a poorly combined meal so that the body has to expend a lot of energy and time in trying to sort out the mess in the stomach. The result is, of course, lack of energy. One of the most immediate benefits of correct food-combining is the increase in energy levels. You wake up feeling rested and refreshed, never groggy or listless. If you have any digestive problems, allergies, or suffer from a lack of energy, the best thing you could do is to try combining your foods correctly, for at least a month. I'll guarantee that you will never go back to a badly combined meal again; it is just not worth it. (Well, you may, but you'll be back on track soon enough.)

Food-combining is just common sense when you get down to it. You may find, for example, that you can eat certain foods together that may cause discomfort in others (this could be dependent on the quantity of food you eat and the efficiency of your digestive tract), but even if you notice no difference in digestive comfort you should notice a huge difference in energy levels.

Implementing Food-Combining

Now that you know what food-combining is, how do you go about implementing it in your diet? Remember the basic guideline—try not to eat a concentrated carbohydrate or starch with a concentrated protein. You can, however, eat salads or non-starchy vegetables with either of these groups. So if you wanted a sandwich, potatoes, corn, pasta, or rice for a meal, you should not eat a protein such as stronger-flavored cheeses (which are higher in protein than the milder flavors), eggs, fish, chicken, meat, or nuts with it. And if you wanted fish, for example, you should omit starch from the meal. Remember that you can always have a fresh salad or steamed fresh vegetables with either a starch or a protein meal.

This can all be very confusing, so let's take it meal by meal.

BREAKFAST

This should preferably consist of fresh, seasonal fruit. Remember, fruit is the ideal first food of the day and you should try to eat at least one fruit meal daily. It is a good idea to have your fruit meal at breakfast simply because you should try to put as little strain on digestion as possible after the body's rigorous cleansing activities of the night before.

Summer fruits, such as grapes, are available up to autumn or fall, but most fruits overlap at the beginning and the end of the seasons. Bananas, pineapples, and passion fruit (granadilla) are available throughout the year without needing to be put into cold storage. Winter fruits such as apples and oranges are often available in summer as they keep well, but fruit that has been in cold storage is not nearly as tasty as fruit in season, and the cores are often black. We try not to eat fruit that is out of season as we don't enjoy it as much when its season eventually comes around. Take apples, for example. Although they are available throughout the year, we eat them in the wintertime so that by the end of summer, we look forward to some fresh, crunchy apples and we enjoy them more. Also, apples that have been in cold storage tend to be floury.

Here is a simple guide to the seasonal fruits:

Summer Fruits:
- Apricots
- Bananas
- Cherries
- Grapes
- Litchis
- Mangoes
- Peaches
- Pineapples
- Plums
- Prunes
- Strawberries and all berries
- Watermelons

Winter Fruits:
- Apples
- Bananas
- Grapefruit
- Guavas
- Kiwi
- Minneola
- Oranges
- Papaya
- Pears
- Pineapples
- Tangerines

Fruit can be eaten whole, chopped in fruit salads, or blended in fruit shakes and smoothies. Although the best way to eat fruit is in its whole state, sometimes it makes the meal just a bit more interesting to have a salad or a shake. (To make fruit shakes, blend correctly combined fruit [see food-combining chart on page 266] in a food processor.) One of our favorite blends in summer is mangoes with pineapple, but any combination can be delicious. Another is our cashew shake or smoothie, which consists of raw cashews with fresh pineapple, frozen berries, and freshly squeezed orange juice (see recipe section for quantities). When making a fruit shake, raisins or dates can be added to a sub-acid or sweet fruit combination for extra flavor. Another great idea is apples and bananas with a teaspoon of macerated (mashed) dates dissolved in warm water. Nuts can be added to any acid or sub-acid fruit shake.

Acid/Sub-Acid/Sweet Fruits:

Now what is all this talk about acid, sub-acid, and sweet fruits? Most people find that certain fruits do not digest comfortably with others and this is simply because of the fruit's nutrient structures. For example, sweet fruits have very high sugar content and are digested like starches, whereas acid fruits are digested in a similar way to proteins. You may find you feel fine when you mix different fruits together that I suggest are difficult to digest. Listening to your body is more important than food-combining, so keep in mind if you are comfortable and benefit from mixing oranges and bananas, then do it. Here are some examples of the different fruits and their groupings:

Acid Fruit	Sub-Acid Fruit	Sweet Fruit
Gooseberries	Apples	Bananas
Grapefruit	Apricots	Dates
Guavas	Berries	Dried fruit
Kiwi	Cherries	Figs
Kumquats	Grapes	Papaya
Lemons	Litchis	Papino
Limes	Loquats	Persimmons
Melons	Mangoes	Prunes
Oranges	Nectarines	Raisins
Pineapples	Peaches	Seedless Grapes
Passion Fruit	Pears	Sultanas (Unbleached)
Pomegranates	Plums	
Quinces	Prickly Pears	
Strawberries		
Tangerines		
Watermelon		

Acid fruits combine well with sub-acid fruits; sweet fruits combine well with sub-acid fruits; and sub-acid fruits combine well with both other groups. When eating fruits from two incompatible groups, it is best to separate these fruits by at least an hour.

If you find it difficult at first to have fruit for breakfast, start by adding a piece of sweet fruit to a starch breakfast. An example would be oats with raisins and banana. Sweet fruits and starches digest in a similar pH environment in the stomach, although fruit takes less time. As a transitional meal, this combination can be eaten in the beginning. Fruit on its own is best, so make this your ultimate aim.

MID-MORNING SNACK

An ideal mid-morning snack would be more fresh fruit. But if you battle with this in the beginning, a slice of fresh whole wheat toast with butter and/or avocado or any other salad topping suffices as a transitional snack.

LUNCH

Lunch could be more fruit if you liked, or a fresh salad with a starch or a protein. (See the food-combining chart on page 265 and the recipes in chapter eighteen.) You might like to try a fresh salad containing tomatoes, lettuce, and cucumbers with any non-starch vegetables such as broccoli, mushrooms, and carrots (some vegetables such as carrots and pumpkin do contain more starch than others but they still digest well as a neutral vegetable with either protein or starch), peas, or cauliflower. These are also referred to as neutral vegetables in the food-combining chart at the back of this book. You might want to add one type of starch, such as baked potatoes or whole wheat bread, to this. You might prefer to add one type of protein, such as fish, to the meal rather than a starch. It is also best not to mix two types of starch or protein at a meal as each type digests far more easily on its own. Also, when we eat more than one type per meal, we tend to overeat.

If you have opted for a light lunch, you might need a mid-afternoon snack, but wait at least three hours after lunch if you had starch or protein, or one to two hours afterward if you ate a salad or some fruit. A portion of fruit is the ideal snack.

DINNER

Dinner could be the same as lunch, but if you had protein in the day you should not eat another portion of protein for supper. Protein should ideally not be eaten more than once a day and neither should starch unless you are a very active athlete or an active child. Remember to include half a cup of raw, unsalted nuts at least three times a week if you are a vegetarian, as many nuts and seeds contain as much protein as fish. It's also a good idea to include an avocado a day as this will prevent any cravings for fatty or oily food. In fact, if you ever crave fatty foods, eating avocados or nuts will satisfy that craving quite easily as the craving usually indicates a lack of essential fatty acids, found abundantly in these foods.

It is not a good idea to eat after supper as the digestion tends to be less efficient toward the end of the day, especially after sunset. It is also not a good idea to go to bed with food in your stomach. Most cooked meals take about four hours to digest, and as the body needs to focus its energy and attention on any healing and repair that need to be done while you sleep, your last meal of the day should be eaten at least three hours before you retire.

Bear in mind that digestion depends on many factors, such as how much you eat and what emotional state you are in. If relaxed, the body takes far less time to digest food, but if you are worked up, stressed, or upset about anything it can take a lot longer. A poorly combined meal can take from four to eight hours and sometimes even longer to digest, depending on the condition of your stomach.

Follow the times generally taken for food to digest:

- Fruit properly combined—fifteen minutes to two hours
- Fruit badly combined—up to four hours to leave the stomach and during this time it will repeat on you
- Fresh salad with no dressing—one to two hours
- Fresh salad with a dressing that contains oil—up to four hours, longer if the oil is not cold-pressed or extra-virgin
- Starch meal with neutral vegetables—two to four hours
- Protein meal with neutral vegetables—two to four hours
- Badly combined starch and protein meal—four to twelve hours

If you still feel uncertain about how to change to the Perfect Health lifestyle, there are various simple programs for you to start with. For more detailed information, see chapters fourteen and sixteen. If you need a day-by-day guide with recipes, motivation, and tips, go to www.100daystohealth.com or www.mary-anns.com. These sites will allow you access to a program that covers just over three months of day-by-day, meal-by-meal recipes and support for following Perfect Health.

OPTIONS TO CHOOSE FROM

Option 1

Start your day with properly combined fruit and eat as much of it as you like throughout the morning if you are still hungry. Try not to eat fruit with any other food as this combination will ferment in the stomach and cause digestive problems. The one exception is raw nuts and seeds eaten with acid and sub-acid fruit, which helps those who feel they need a more substantial meal or those with blood sugar problems.

Try not to drink tea or coffee during the morning, or try at least to cut back on your intake to start with. Tea and coffee contain both tannin and caffeine, substances that are toxic to the body. Many people who suddenly cut these beverages out of their diets often suffer from withdrawal, experiencing unpleasant symptoms such as headaches, nausea, irritability, sleeplessness, and the shakes. If you are a regular tea or coffee drinker, start off by reducing your intake gradually. Caffeine can result in insomnia and lumps in the breasts, and it is also potentially harmful to the human fetus. Caffeine is also known to upset that very important endocrine system that controls every function in the body, including reproduction. I have known quite a few women who have battled to conceive and then within a few months of stopping their one cup of coffee a day became pregnant. This is a huge issue in a country such as America, where coffee is so readily available. Remember that caffeine is a stimulant that affects the central nervous system, hormones, the heart, and the kidneys. You may find yourself very comfortable with a good decaffeinated version and most good coffee shops use coffee that has been decaffeinated using steam and water, not chemicals.

Tannin is less toxic but is suspected of causing liver damage in regular large quantities. It is best to drink a glass of filtered water, fresh fruit juice, or an herb or fruit tea when you are thirsty. There are also cereal drinks and carob alternatives to coffee, tea, and hot chocolate.

Stop eating fruit an hour before lunch to give your stomach a chance to clear. For lunch, have a large fresh salad or a selection of raw vegetables with hummus, or an avocado dip such as guacamole if a salad seems too complicated. (Include one type of starch here if still hungry.) You can follow the salad with a protein or starch if you like.

If you need an afternoon snack, try one or two pieces of fruit or a handful of preservative-free dried fruit.

For supper start with a large raw salad. Include one type of protein or starch (not to be eaten together) and as many steamed vegetables as you like. Try to eat animal protein no more than three times a week, if you can.

Dr. Richard Wurtman, a well-known nutrition researcher, has found that protein may be better eaten during the day, for example, at lunch; this is because protein appears to stimulate the brain. Starches are best at night because they appear to raise our serotonin levels, making us feel relaxed, happy, and sleepy. Listen to your body and see what works for you.

Option 2

Eat as much properly combined fruit and vegetables throughout the day as you like, making sure you eat at least three to four pieces of fruit a day to stop any sugar cravings. Include half a cup of raw nuts or seeds a day. Listen to your body, not to your taste buds. Do not eat if you are not hungry. Make sure to leave at least one hour before supper. For dinner, follow the suggestions in Option 1.

Option 3

Eat fruit at every meal and whenever you are hungry. Half a cup of nuts (not groundnuts, as these are heated legumes, which are more difficult to digest), unsalted and unroasted, should be eaten at least three times a week. Remember to eat a wide variety of in-season fruit. Nuts are best eaten either with a salad or with acid fruits (see food-combining chart for fruits on page 266). Avocados should also be included for the days you don't eat nuts. Eat one per day if you are watching your weight, but if not, three to four can be easily managed.

This is a totally raw diet and one I recommend for a process of detoxification, or for people who like the idea of living on a totally raw diet. (No, you don't have to, but some like to!)

This is also the diet I recommend if you have serious diseases such as cancer, heart disease, AIDS, or any autoimmune diseases. We have seen remarkable improvements in thousands of people over the years on this strict, raw diet and have one lovely lady who fully recovered from liver cancer and now twelve years later is considered cured. Many others with Lupus, multiple sclerosis, ME (Yuppie Flu), high blood pressure, and even diabetes have seen a dramatic turn in their health. It is best to be monitored by a natural health consultant. (See www.mary-anns.com for a complete list of people who can help you.)

Our family lived like this for six months and we were in exceptional health. It made us become quite anti-social, and I had to help the children cope in the real world. We now follow Option 2 most of the time and only follow Option 3 for a week or two every few months, especially at the change of the seasons.

If you ever feel a flu or cold coming on, immediately start this 100 percent raw program and within twelve to twenty-four hours you will see a huge improvement in your health.

Option 4

This is a combination of the previous three options that can be alternated on a daily basis. Whatever you do, try to have at least one meal a day that consists entirely of fruit with some nuts or seeds if possible.

There is no need to weigh or measure your food; you must listen to your body and eat until you are satisfied. In the beginning you may find yourself or your children gorging on fruit—don't panic or try and hold back; your body is trying to correct the nutritional imbalances that have developed over the years and within a few days to a few months, your appetites will calm down. I clearly remember one day eating eight mangoes, and another day I ate 4 pounds of fresh dates! Did I mention that I was a compulsive overeater as well as a sugarholic? Within a few months my appetite calmed down and as much as I have a healthy appetite it is no longer out of control. Your body will correct these problems—just give it time and enjoy yourself. Today if I eat two dates in a month, it is a lot. I find them far too sweet and prefer combining them with coconut. (See recipes.)

So there we are. Changing to the Perfect Health lifestyle is not nearly as complicated as you may have feared. At this stage, ask yourself if you suffer from any of the symptoms I have mentioned: indigestion, spastic colon, allergies, lack of energy, or any other digestive problems. If you do, you have everything to gain and nothing to lose (except maybe excess weight) if you combine your food correctly. If you are still unsure, try one of these simple programs for two weeks and then you will have all the proof you need! Remember, if you need a day-by-day program, log on to www.100daystohealth.com.

CHAPTER FIVE

Foods and Moods
Your Food and How It Affects Your Moods, Behavior, and Mental Health

I WAS SPEAKING TO MARGARET, a friend of mine, the other day. She has a degree in social work, specializing in psychology, and has worked at one of the top crisis centers in her country for many years. "Mary-Ann," she said, "in all my years of counseling, I've reached the conclusion that 99 percent of all mental and emotional problems are directly related to the way that people eat and live." She added that she had yet to come across an individual who was glowing with vitality and health when he or she came for counseling. The old maxim, you *are* what you eat, has never been more apt than it is today.

We've all moved so far from our natural lifestyles that it is hardly surprising that people have the problems they do. For example, take a look at the high-fat diet, which most Western societies consume. This can result in a mild form of depression or a pessimistic outlook on life, and then there is the very real risk of cancer! Fat, which is the most complex of foods to break down, results in more blood than normal being diverted from the brain. When body activity and energy are focused on the stomach, which is what happens when too much fat is consumed, the brain does not receive enough oxygen and we become listless and apathetic, our mental processes become slow and confused, and mild depression sets in. On the other hand, essential fats are needed for the brain just to function on a day-to-day level; deficiency of the right fats can result in mental sluggishness. (See chapter eight.)

At the opposite end of the scale, drastic dieting is another common problem today, and it can have devastating effects on the nervous system and often poses serious health risks. One of the main reasons for this is that carbohydrates and fats are usually cut out completely or cut down drastically in most diets. Carbohydrates convert to natural glucose, which is the primary nutrient needed for the maintenance of a healthy nervous system. Often the first sign of this deficiency is the extreme irritability that most dieters suffer.

Another harmful practice that many diets encourage is the consumption of foods or substances that are extremely low in calories but high in artificial additives. Although this may result in rapid weight loss, it can leave the dieter feeling quite terrible and may even cause long-term health problems (see chapter nine). These types of diets discourage the dieter from eating such foods as avocados, bananas, dates, and raisins, all of which satisfy many nutritional needs and promote mental and emotional health. It makes absolutely no sense to be allowed relative freedom to consume quantities of low-calorie diet sodas laced with artificial flavorings, artificial colorants, and artificial sweeteners (all of which can cause irritability, depression, and confusion) while being discouraged from consuming the foods that God intended us to eat.

High-protein diets have been found to affect the mind and emotions negatively. This type of diet can result in metabolic disturbances, mental confusion, lack of ability to control emotions, and liver and kidney damage. Apparently the ancient Chinese placed their prisoners on a high-protein diet so as to cause a breakdown in emotional resolve and mental health! High-protein diets are known to affect the thyroid gland, which controls mental clarity. You may lose weight on a high-protein diet but you can also lose your mind!

Another common dietary mistake is the consumption of refined foods. Processed sugars and grains especially deplete the body of the vital B complex vitamins. The reason for this is simple. The body needs vitamin B complex to assimilate sugar but this vitamin is removed or destroyed during processing, resulting in the body robbing itself of the vitamin B it requires. As vitamin B is the anti-stress vitamin, we then find that we cannot cope very well with stress without it. Eating refined foods can also lead to hyperactivity and hypoglycemia, with the following symptoms: confusion, forgetfulness, poor concentration, emotional outbursts, quick-temperedness, irritability, impatience, depression, weepiness, bad vision (double or blurred), sensitivity to bright light, fatigue, sleeplessness, cold sweats, blackouts, headaches, joint pains, muscle cramps, and cravings for sweets and coffee.

You would think that these alarming symptoms, of which there are many sufferers (at least 50 percent of all women who have been to see me suffer from many of these ailments), would be sufficient to ban refined sugars and grains, together with their products.

Hypoglycemia also contributes to bad behavior because it can result in aggression. With hypoglycemia, the higher, less primitive area of the brain cannot work efficiently as the brain requires sufficient glucose to work properly; when these socially responsible areas of the brain shut down because of lack of energy, aberrant behavior results. This may result in aggression, irritability, confusion, amnesia, depression, and many other psychological disorders such as neurosis, psychosis, or schizophrenia.

Refined sugar and alcohol have a similar effect on blood sugar levels in that both raise blood sugar very fast. The body then reacts (basically to save your life as high blood sugar can put you into a diabetic coma from which you could die) and the pancreas goes into overdrive to produce insulin and down your blood sugar comes. Over time this usually results in low blood sugar or hypoglycemia.

This would explain the violent behavior that results when some people consume alcohol or even just refined sugar. It certainly explained my behavior and the behavior of many people I have dealt with over the years.

The choice is ours. I am certain of one thing, and I have seen it over and over again: all these symptoms can be cured completely by steering clear of refined sugars, starches, and alcohol and by changing one's eating habits to include quantities of fresh fruit and vegetables in the diet. I used to suffer from all the above symptoms and at times became quite suicidal. I thought that I had inherited the depression problems from my father's side of the family. Little did I realize that as health-conscious as I was, the one sweet or chocolate I ate every other day (and at times more often than that) affected my blood sugar levels to such an extent that I would look in the mirror and tell myself that I was mad. If it had not been for my desire to find the answers to my problems, with the guidance that I believe could only come from God, and with the support of an extremely loving and caring husband, I might not be here today to tell you this.

It has been extremely interesting to discover that this problem of fluctuating blood sugar levels, along with the accompanying symptoms and cravings for sweet things, tends to run in families. Frequently, sufferers also have a history of drinking problems, as did my father and my grandfather before him. But the most amazing thing of all was the discovery that by changing to a diet high in fresh, raw fruits, all these symptoms disappeared within a couple of days. I have not suffered from these symptoms for many years, unless I have eaten refined flour or sugar over an extended period of two or three days, which can happen quite easily over Christmas and New Year. As you can see, I am far from perfect, but at least I now know why I sometimes feel the way I do, and that makes it so much easier to deal with any problems when they arise. I have dealt with both sugarholics and alcoholics and both find that when they include plenty of fresh fruit daily by following the first two Perfect Health steps, they don't crave sugar or alcohol anymore. The most dramatic case was a man who lost his business, family, and home due to alcoholism but within three months had them all back after he focused on changing his diet, which included plenty of fresh and preservative-free dried fruit.

Refined Carbohydrates

In 1980 a clinical study appeared in the *American Journal of Clinical Nutrition*, reporting that people who ate too many refined carbohydrates exhibited neurotic tendencies and personality changes. This condition seems particularly to affect adolescents. It was found that the personality changes included sensitivity to criticism, poor impulse control, frequent irritability, hostile behavior, and a tendency to anger easily. It seems that by doing away with refined carbohydrates, we could do away with the generation gap! Other symptoms included sleep disturbance, chronic debilitating fatigue (sounds like Yuppie Flu?) and depression, recurring fevers of unknown origin, abdominal and/or chest pains, and headaches.

Barbara Reed Stitt in her book *Food and Behavior* says:

This lack of blood sugar starves every cell in the body, leading to a general feeling of weakness. But the cells of the brain are specially starved. As the blood sugar drops, the cerebrum—the area of the brain responsible for thought, learning and moral and social behavior—starts to shut down, and the brain diverts its dwindling energy resources to the brain stem, which controls the more primitive responses: the drives for food and sex, aggressive/defensive instincts, basic bodily functions, etc. (40–41).

What makes this particularly frightening is that the cerebrum is only fully developed by age twenty-five and the biggest consumers of refined sugar are under twenty-five years old! Add alcohol to that, which most people under that age consume, and you have a disaster waiting to happen. I know there are emotional issues that have driven teenagers to do crazy things such as commit suicide or shoot their peers at school, but I personally believe these episodes are triggered by refined sugar and alcohol. We are raising a nation of junk-food addicts and then blaming their bad behavior on bullies! Bullies have been around for centuries (think of Goliath), yet only in the last twenty-odd years has teenage behavior become so violent.

It seems to me that if we control the blood sugar of the world by dealing with malnutrition and banning refined sugar we could wipe out criminal behavior and delinquency!

Even if you do not lose your mind when you eat foods containing refined sugar, you may still find in time, depending on your genetic "weak spot," that your body will start to act up. Whether it develops allergies, arthritis, heart disease, cancer, diabetes, or a host of other diseases, sooner or later the body has to pay the price for the way we feed it.

Neal Barnard, M.D., author of *Breaking the Food Seduction*, says:

> Sugar causes the release of opiates in the brain. But that opiate response does more than make you feel good. It also has a marked appetite driving effect. You've experienced it: You had a little bit of an appetite before you took your first bite of sugar. Might taste good, you thought. But once it touches your lips, sugar's opiate effects break through the dam holding back your appetite, and an army of dieticians could not save you from the binge that sweeps you away. Inside your brain, the opiates triggered by the sweet taste are busy resetting all your internal priorities to make you care about one thing and one thing only: eating more of what just passed your lips (33).

Barbara Reed Stitt, author of *Food and Behavior*, believes some people are biochemically predisposed to sugar addiction or cravings, particularly if they have a family history of alcoholism, depression, or obesity. This was definitely the case with me.

Isn't this enough evidence to ban refined carbohydrates from your household? When Mark and I changed to this way of eating, I remember telling my children that I would no longer buy them candy, cookies, or ice cream as I loved them too much to poison them. What about their sense of deprivation, you may ask. Well, the only thing you'll be depriving your children of is any one of the above symptoms. I have seen my daughters grow up and be deprived of premenstrual tension, heavy periods, skin problems, weight issues; although they have tried processed foods, they always come back to the Natural Way because as they say, "It's worth it and it works." In the case of grandparents or friends who insist that they must give them candy to show them they love them, read this chapter to them. In fact, giving children refined sugar is, in my opinion, a form of child abuse! That may sound harsh, but if you are consciously giving your children a substance that has a drug-like effect, can cause depression, suicidal feelings, ill health, mood swings, learning and behavioral problems, and can predispose them toward criminal and delinquent behavior, would you not consider that child abuse? Hopefully reading this chapter will make them realize that your children are definitely not deprived. The kids won't even miss the treats. Just give them sweet alternatives—dried fruits, especially dates and raisins, are ideal. (See recipe section and www.mary-anns.com for plenty of healthy, unrefined sugar-free snacks.)

This is a subject I could write an entire book on. If you think this is a radical approach and you cannot begin to imagine how you or your family's health and mental stability could possibly be affected by diet, try removing it for six weeks and replacing it with loads of fresh and preservative-free dried fruit (follow the first three steps at least). If you see no improvement then go back to your old diet and lifestyle (somehow I know you won't).

Another excellent book to read on this subject is *Sugar Blues* by William Dufty. This will leave you without a doubt as to how harmful refined foods are.

The link between nutrition and emotional well-being does not only include refined carbohydrates. It was found that cow's milk produced the same undesirable behavior just about as frequently as synthetic coloring. Milk has also been found as a cause of enuresis (bed-wetting) in older children. This would no doubt put an emotional and mental strain not only on the child but on the parents as well. (There is more about milk in chapter six.)

Shortages or deficiencies in vitamins and minerals can also result in mental and emotional problems. Low iron levels can result in impaired judgment and reasoning, and low zinc levels can contribute to anorexia, bulimia, and a craving for salt and sugar. Milk is a cause of both iron and zinc deficiencies. Taking supplements is not the answer. These are inorganic, artificial substances that the body cannot metabolize fully. The answer is to eat a diet high in raw food (at least 75–80 percent). This way you ensure that you are getting the maximum amount of nutrients and by combining your food properly, you will get the maximum break-down and absorption of these nutrients. If you feel the need to take in extra nutrients then purchase a good quality juice extractor and extract the juice of organic dark green leafy vegetables (barley grass juice is best and wheat grass is good, as well) and the juice of red, orange, or yellow fruit and vegetables such as carrots and beets. If this is too much like hard work, you can use the dried organic barley, carrot, and beet juices available at the market. (Check out www.mary-anns.com for the ones I use and recommend.)

Dr. F. M. Pottenger conducted some fascinating experiments, initially on cats, to determine the disadvantages of eating cooked food. The results of these experiments are documented in his book, *Pottenger's Cats.* The experiments revealed that cats fed a totally cooked diet of meat, cod-liver oil, and pasteurized milk became irritable. The females became increasingly aggressive, while the males became more docile and their interest in sex slackened or became perverted by abnormal sexual activities. On the other hand, cats eating exactly the same food, but in its raw state, were in peak condition with none of the above behavioral abnormalities being exhibited. Dr. Pottenger then went on to use his *raw food therapy* on humans with tremendous success.

I know that when we enter a very stressful period at work (usually traveling around the world and doing two talks a day), Mark and I both go on a total raw food (fresh fruit, vegetables, nuts, seeds, and avocado) program as we find we are calmer, more clear-headed, and able to get by on very little sleep without any detrimental effects. Unfortunately what most of us do is eat badly when under stress, which only exacerbates the problem.

When food is cooked, many nutrients are either partially or totally destroyed. The water-soluble vitamins B and C are especially vulnerable and are destroyed in foods which are cooked in water, as are the fat-soluble vitamins A, D, E, and K when food is fried. Cooking also changes the structure of certain nutrients, resulting in difficulty in assimilation by the body. For this reason, it is best to steam any foods that you might want cooked as this method tends to destroy the least nutrients.

Caffeine

Caffeine is another substance found in our food that can affect the way our brain works. I have heard from countless people who find that their moods and stress levels improve dramatically after removing caffeine from their diets. Jason, our son-in-law, found that he tended to become quite aggressive in most circumstances. His diet had improved dramatically when he married our daughter Melissa (he had no choice!). During the first year of marriage he had reduced his coffee intake down to just a cup a day, but it was only when he decided he could live without that one cup that his aggressive nature disappeared completely. He is now one of the calmest and gentlest people I know!

Because caffeine is so structurally similar to adenosine, it binds to nerve-cell receptors in place of adenosine, and in so doing prevents the adenosine from binding there. Adenosine is an important regulator of body processes, particularly nerves' transmission signals, and has a calming effect on the body. Injections of adenosine or substances that increase adenosine levels can cause lethargy and sleep. Adenosine can also dilate blood vessels and slow down gastrointestinal motility, protect against seizures, retard the body's reaction to stress, and lower heart rate, blood pressure, and body temperature.

When caffeine binds to these nerve cell sites the nerve cells fire more rapidly, which in turn affects the brain and central nervous and cardiovascular systems. This has the opposite effect that adenosine does and places enormous stress on the body. Panic attacks, nervousness, poor sleep patterns, and irritability are a few of the problems that can result from this reaction. There is some research indicating that the sudden death by heart failure that occurs on the sports field is related to caffeine consumption.

The central nervous system is directly linked to endocrine function and affects everything in the body. Caffeine also has a direct effect on the blood sugar levels as it affects the adrenal glands. This can, in turn, contribute to high and low blood sugar and blood pressure problems.

If you do drink or eat beverages or food containing caffeine, make sure you don't do so before a medical examination as you could end up leaving with a prescription for blood sugar or blood pressure problems. I have yet to meet a doctor who asks a patient whether they have had caffeine two to three hours before the consultation.

How much caffeine will affect you? Well, no one really knows; some people are adversely affected from one cup of tea daily, others seem immune drinking six-plus cups of coffee a day. At the end of the day, long-term ingestion of caffeine, even in small quantities, can affect you.

I suggest you start replacing caffeinated drinks with caffeine-free herb or fruit teas. Replace caffeinated sodas with natural sugar and preservative-free drinks and replace chocolate with carob bars.

RECAP

What kind of diet encourages mental and emotional well-being?

- A diet that supplies all the necessary nutrients and is whole and unprocessed
- A diet that is free from non foods or refined junk foods that will rob the body of nutrients
- A diet that is free from toxic substances such as alcohol, cigarettes, caffeine, and artificial additives and flavorings
- A diet that is high in raw fruit and vegetable content and therefore alkaline-forming

If you follow the Perfect Health program as outlined in this book, you will be sure that your diet encompasses all the above criteria. And you will experience not only mental and emotional well-being, but the physical well-being that goes with it. You will be in control of your mind and emotions and the improvement in your overall quality of life will be worth the small sacrifices and discipline involved.

Here are two of the many people who have benefited from the principles outlined in this chapter:

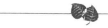

Hi Mary-Ann,
I just returned from my monthly appointment with my psychiatrist, and couldn't wait to write to you.

Last month, I gave her a copy of Perfect Health and told her that it was her turn to do some homework. Today, she reported back to me that she loved the book, has altered her family's entire diet, and is referring loads of her patients to your book! I am so excited! She commented several times about how much better I am doing—all around (looking good and feeling good).

From what I understand, she is one of the better psychiatrists in my city, and if we have her on board, I can only assume that she will spread the word to her colleagues! People's lives are going to change! I just wanted to share.
Cyndi

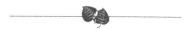

Hi Mary-Ann,
I hit my all-time low in self-respect in 2001 when I hit my all-time high on the scale at nearly 200 pounds. I felt worthless and alone even though people surrounded me. No one could understand my obsession with my weight and subsequently my obsession with food. I thought about food all the time. I remember days where I would sit and pray for God to help me think about something else. I felt ugly.

What upset me most was I knew why I was overweight, I just did not know how to fix it. I felt like a bad Christian, a hypocrite. I had lost control of my body; I no longer knew how to read the signs. I ate because it tasted good and eating made me feel better for a short moment. I had come to realize that I was no better than a drunk or a drug addict and if God could help those people as I had seen Him do before then He could help me, too.

So I decided to confess; I told my husband about my secret life— the life where I would eat small amounts in public and huge amounts when no one was around. But why did I do this? Years of incorrect food choices and simply being overweight turned my life into a vicious cycle of feeling bad and making more bad food choices. My life was ruled by the diet world, any diet I could get my hands on. The very same people who try to guide us put huge restrictions on our lives: no carbohydrates, no protein, and no starch. They give us strict formulas and diets, so instead of getting to the root of our problem we are left thinking about food all day, planning breakfast, planning lunch, and planning supper and not listening to our bodies like we should.

So I threw away all my diets and started to tune into my body while following the Natural Way. I instantly felt better. I prayed for God's help and He held my hand the whole way. Making the correct food choices, I prayed for God to bless the food for my body; how could I have asked Him to bless a chocolate for my body?

I lost 30 pounds in seven months with no diets—just correct food choices and listening to my body. I no longer felt insecure, I could walk into a room and hear people laughing and not worry that they were laughing at me.

And then I found out I was pregnant. Well, now I was even more determined not to pick up excess weight. I had progressed from the old me that would find any excuse to put on my "winter coat" for protection. My body is God's temple and now it was to be a baby-making factory. I gained 20 pounds during my pregnancy and had lost them four days after I had my son. I breast-fed and lost 15 more pounds over the next few months. My weight has stabilized and the last time I weighed so little was when I was sixteen years old! My son is one this week, and I am a very happy, healthy mommy with a happy, healthy boy. I have God to thank for His unconditional support and guidance and you to thank for your knowledge and guidance.

Being a devout Christian, I believe that nothing happens without a reason. God has a purpose with everything that happens in my life. The opportunity to learn about the Natural Way lifestyle was one of the best things that happened to me in my life.
Lauren

CHAPTER SIX

Got Milk? Get Sick!
Calcium, Osteoporosis, and Dairy Products: Is There a Connection?

THE CONNECTION between calcium and dairy products is something that had confused me for many years. First, I discovered that whenever I ate or drank any dairy products, especially milk, I would get a terrific buildup of mucus and I seemed to be spending my life clearing my throat or blowing my nose. I also discovered that when I discontinued the dairy products, within a couple of days the mucus would be gone. The same can be said for all three of my daughters. Melissa's tonsillitis would clear up, Marie-Claire's nose would stop running, and Meredith's ear infection would clear up—until I introduced the dairy products again.

Now you might ask, how could I have been so stupid? Well, it was quite simple. I believed all the old wives' tales about calcium and dairy products. You know the sort: "Your children's bones will crumble"; "You can't cut dairy products out of your diet or you'll suffer from osteoporosis" (brittle bones due to the loss of minerals, especially calcium). Yet I kept coming across an article or a book telling me that I'd be far better off if I cut dairy out of my diet completely. So I decided to investigate.

What did those people advocating dairy products have to gain? Well, it made economic sense for the dairy industry to wax lyrical about the tremendous health benefits of consuming their products. And then there were certain members of the medical profession who got quite worked up about the need for dairy products in the diet. Perhaps they were just misguided, or perhaps they saw themselves losing a lot of revenue from those poor people suffering from ear infections, tonsillitis, asthma, and sinusitis.

Then I looked at those suggesting that I eliminate dairy products from my diet. What did they have to gain? Nothing! I wasn't being sold a special supplement to make up for all the calcium that I wouldn't get from milk, and they weren't getting any business from my family as we were no longer sick.

But the bearers of bad news did not stop. Regardless of the fact that my children never had the slightest sniffle and were pictures of glowing health, the comments came fast and furiously: "My doctor says you'll all get rickets." (Rickets, by the way, is due to a lack of vitamin D or sunshine rather than lack of calcium.) "My sister-in-law is a dietitian and she says your children won't grow properly." (After discontinuing dairy products for years, all three of my girls are in the top 10 percent for their height.) The best was when Melissa came home from school one day to tell me, "Mommy, my health teacher says I'll get holes in my teeth if I don't drink milk, and I'm the only one in the class without any fillings!"

So what are the facts? It's a fact that the countries that have the highest incidence of dental decay (which, by the way, is classed as a disease) and osteoporosis also have the highest intake of dairy products. In countries with the lowest intake of dairy products there is also the lowest incidence of these diseases. I have also seen that many of the women who seek help from me, regardless of the fact that they take in vast quantities of dairy products, have been unable to stop the loss of calcium from their bones.

It should be quite obvious that dairy products will not prevent the body from losing calcium, nor will it cure calcium deficiencies. Why? Well, to start with, we need the correct calcium-to-phosphorus ratio to be able to use calcium efficiently, and the best ratio in foods for optimum use is found in dark green leafy vegetables. There is way too much phosphorus in milk for us to be able to actually utilize any of the calcium in cow's milk and some research indicates the high phosphorus levels in cow's milk and its products (cheese and yogurt) actually contribute to loss of calcium in our bones. Also, at the age of two or three, when we have most of our teeth, we stop secreting an enzyme called lactase that breaks down the sugar in milk. This indicates clearly that we are designed to be weaned at this age. As Dr. Marius Barnard (brother of the famed heart surgeon, Dr. Chris Barnard) said at a convention held at Sun City on May 18, 1989, "Humans must be the only mammals who continue to provide milk in their diet after being weaned," and "Man has become a walking disaster because we eat like pigs!"

We also don't secrete the enzyme that breaks down the protein in cow's milk. Calves have this enzyme—it's called rennin. This brings me to another point about milk: cow's milk is perfectly designed for calves and human milk is perfectly designed for humans.

We seem obsessed with getting some kind of milk after our biological weaning age, even though there is absolutely no physiological need for milk in any shape or form. I am continually asked if soy, rice, or goat's milk is a better option. Let me get one thing clear: we do not need any kind of milk, the body does not need it, you are not going to die without it, and in fact, your bones and health will be stronger by not using milk of any kind at all!

Soy Milk

There seems to be research indicating that the daily consumption of soy products can upset your thyroid gland. Look at how many children become constipated using soy milk as a replacement for mother's milk! The thyroid controls many bodily functions, such as the bowels, mental clarity, skin, weight, etc. A baby is designed to be fed by his or her mother for at least the first two years of his or her life. If for any reason you cannot breast-feed (and please find a breast-feeding counselor or organization such as the La Leche League before you give up as there is absolutely no equivalent to breast milk), then goat's milk is a better option than cow, soy, or rice milk. It does not matter who formulated the milk and how many vitamins were added, it is still a huge strain, as a baby was only designed for breast milk. Producing lactose-free milk is no solution as lactose is not the main problem. The main cause is one of the twenty-five protein fractions found in cow's milk and one of them is now known to cause juvenile diabetes. This is probably why diabetes is on the rise in the U.S. as we now have a nation of children raised on cow's milk and encouraged to drink it in large quantities. The stereotype of a good American mother is one that hands her child a plate of cookies and a glass of milk as he or she enters the kitchen. There is now so much research indicating just how harmful cow's milk is that I believe in years to come the dairy industry will be sued for promoting a product as essential when in fact it causes untold misery and ill health! To quote from Dr. Colin Campbell in his book *The China Study*, "Cow's milk may cause one of the most devastating diseases that can befall a child" (*The China Study* 187). There is also research indicating that cow's milk is a major factor in autoimmune diseases such as multiple sclerosis.

Rice Milk

Rice milk is one of those products referred to as junk food sold as health food as it is processed by adding oil, sweetener, and flavors. If you cannot cope without milk as an adult or want to know what to use in your child's cereal, here are a few more natural, less harmful options:

- Blend a ripe banana in a blender with filtered water until rich and creamy and pour this banana milk over cereal
- Use freshly extracted grape or apple juice or a store-bought variety that has no added sugar or preservatives and is 100 percent pure
- If you need milk for your coffee (and hopefully by now it is decaf) the odd bit of cow's milk may be okay, but if you have the option, goat's milk is better. Or if using soy milk, use one that is 100 percent pure with no added oils, fats, flavor, or other products

Other Dairy Products

Cheese, on the other hand, can really be a tough food to exclude, as it appears that it is high in natural opiates known as casomorphins, which are addictive substances that make us want more. No wonder most people are addicted to cheese!

What about yogurt? We have long been told it is an extremely healthy food and we should be including it as part of our daily calcium intake. Well, yes, it is high in calcium, just as milk and cheese are, but it is equally high in phosphorus, making it acid-forming and therefore a substance that will contribute to loss of calcium. If you need to reintroduce the friendly intestinal flora for any reason, then you are better off taking a good quality capsule containing those friendly bacteria; you do not need a whole bunch of mucus-forming, diabetes-promoting, addictive proteins to come into the body together with the friendly bacteria.

So, you may well still be asking, from where are we going to get our calcium? Well, from the food that we as humans were designed to eat— fruits, vegetables, nuts, and seeds. According to any reliable nutritional chart, every single fruit, vegetable, nut, and seed contains calcium (refer to charts at the back of the book). Grains also contain calcium but some of them such as wheat contain phytic acid that tends to bind the calcium.

According to *Fruit for Thought* by Professor B. J. Meyer, a fruitarian diet can supply the daily recommended calcium requirements.

Now, the aim of this book is not to convert everyone to fruitarianism (although many of you would be far better off!) but to make you aware of the very important role that fresh fruit should play in your diet, and to demonstrate that cow's milk is not vital to your health. The recent research completed by Cornell University together with the aid of Chinese researchers and Oxford University shows that dairy calcium is not needed to prevent osteoporosis. The research involved the dietary lifestyles of thousands of Chinese who consume no dairy products whatsoever. According to Dr. Campbell, who headed the project, sufficient calcium is obtained from the vegetables and grains that make up the bulk of their diet. Osteoporosis is uncommon in China and so is dental decay. However, when the Chinese live in America they succumb to dental decay and brittle bones.

Does this mean never eating a slice of cheese or cheesecake again? Absolutely not! But at least now if you or your children suffer from tonsillitis, sinusitis, ear infections, bronchitis, menstrual disorders, or post-nasal drips you know what you need to do; get rid of the dairy for at least three to six weeks, then only occasionally eat it. You will have to see what your body can handle. I had my tonsils out at age four, which got rid of the tonsillitis (the first line of defense in your body are the tonsils by the way) but did not get rid of the problem that then became a post-nasal drip and in my teenage years sinusitis and then very heavy menstrual periods with bad premenstrual tension. When I removed dairy from my diet all these symptoms disappeared and as a bonus so did my cellulite. What a trade-off! Do I ever eat cheese? Yes, if it is put in front of me in a salad, for example, but I may have to clear my throat for the next twenty-four hours. Cheese is no longer one of our daily food groups and all of us are better off for it.

Mark appeared not to be dairy intolerant until we removed dairy from our diets, and then his snoring disappeared and it reappears when he has any dairy, so he also tries to avoid it. He has also found in recent years that an old knee injury flares up when eating cheese, yogurt, or milk, and we have both found that we develop backaches when we regularly consume dairy.

Remember that if any member of your family suffers from mucus-related symptoms or diseases, the best thing you can do is eliminate all dairy products from the diet. You will never suffer from calcium deficiency if you follow the guidelines set out above.

If for some reason you are not too confident about eliminating dairy products from your Perfect Health program, have your blood tested regularly. This way you will be able to monitor your calcium levels and enjoy peace of mind!

Now the question still remains: why do we suffer from such a high incidence of osteoporosis and dental decay? Does milk cause it? Not necessarily, although it could be a contributing factor. One of the main reasons that our systems lose calcium is because of our high acid-forming diet. Certain foods, such as all animal products and, to a lesser degree, all grains, have an acidic reaction on our blood. In other words, meat, chicken, fish, eggs, milk, cheese, yogurt, wheat, rice, corn, and barley are all acid-forming or leave an acid ash or acid minerals such as phosphorus and sulfur in the bloodstream. When our diet is more than 25 percent acid-forming, the body needs to neutralize the acidity in some way. The reason it has to do this is that the blood is slightly alkaline (± 7.35–7.45 on the pH scale) and if the blood were to become acidic, we would die. Rather than allow this to happen, the body utilizes its neutralizer or buffer system, and the main ingredient of this buffer system happens to be the mineral calcium. How does the body obtain calcium? It draws it from its storage place, the bones and teeth, resulting in dental decay and osteoporosis. Way back in 1974, Anand and Linkswiler showed that a high-protein intake resulted in the body losing calcium, and that a low-protein intake facilitated calcium retention. A high-protein diet is an acid-forming diet and will encourage your body to draw calcium out of your bones and teeth, yet another good reason not to embark on a high-protein diet. But your diet does not have to be high-protein to be acid-forming; even a typical high-grain or processed vegetarian diet can be acid-forming. Remember that many other habits are also acid-forming, such as cigarette smoking, drinking alcohol, and the use of drugs (including most kinds of medication).

Let's take a look at the average Westerner's way of eating, and how this affects calcium levels:

- Wake up—tea or coffee with milk and sugar. All are acid-forming! Even if you are health-conscious and drink a cereal beverage (a tea or coffee replacement made from grains or cereals like barley or wheat) it is also acid-forming
- Breakfast—this usually consists of either one or all the following: pancakes, waffles, bagels, toast, bacon and eggs, cereal, cooked porridge, muesli, French toast, toasted sandwich. All are acid-forming! Fruit is sometimes eaten with these foods and although fresh, uncooked fruit is normally alkaline-forming, when eaten with other foods it tends to ferment in the stomach, causing acidity. Add another cup of coffee and you have another acid-forming substance
- Mid-morning snack—sandwiches, cookies, candy, chocolate, tea, or coffee; all are acid-forming
- Lunch—an average non-business meal would consist of sandwiches, margarine, peanut butter, jelly, cheese, tuna, pizza, hotdogs, or hamburgers. All are acid-forming! A bit of salad or a slice of tomato is sometimes included in some lunches. Although all salad and vegetables are alkaline-forming, once you combine your food incorrectly you end up with an acidic mess in your stomach
- Mid-afternoon snack—cookies, coffee, donut, candy, chocolates with tea or coffee. All are acid-forming
- Dinner—meat, chicken or fish, rice, pizza, pies, macaroni and cheese, spaghetti, and maybe a glass of wine. All are acid-forming! Salads and vegetables are often included in this meal and are all alkaline-forming. But this is usually followed by dessert that, in any form, is acid-forming. So too is the last cup of tea and coffee of the day. Add to this cigarette smoke and air pollution, and the acid-forming percentage is pushed up even further

You can see through this example of an average person's daily diet why we have such a high incidence of dental decay and osteoporosis. (Remember that the body uses its own stores of calcium in the teeth and bones to neutralize the acidity to prevent you from dying.)

How do we overcome this problem? Simply by returning to a more natural alkaline-forming diet (one that is at least 75 percent). And the way to achieve this is to:

- Start each day with fresh fruit and to continue eating fruit during the course of the morning when hungry
- With each meal, other than fruit meals, enjoy a large fresh salad with as many other vegetables (raw or steamed) as you can manage
- Make sure that all meals are properly combined
- Try not to eat protein more than once a day and three times a week is even better
- Snack only on fresh or dried fruit or raw vegetables in between meals
- Avoid tea and coffee if possible, or limit to one cup per day

In addition to the Perfect Health five steps, try and exercise daily, as every time your muscles pull on your bones they get stronger. You need a minimum of twenty to thirty minutes a day of regular exercise (see chapter ten), preferably outdoors as natural sunlight on the skin converts cholesterol (lowering cholesterol) into vitamin D, which is essential for the body to be able to use calcium efficiently. To get the cholesterol from the liver where it is processed to the cells where it is needed for this and many other processes, you need to make sure you are taking in natural unsaturated fats. (See chapters eight and ten.) I have found flaxseed oil to be one of the most beneficial unsaturated fats in this instance. Including one to three tablespoons of flaxseed oil or a blend of natural plant oils with a high percentage of flaxseed oil daily in your diet would be of great support in preventing loss of calcium. (Visit www.mary-anns.com for the ones I recommend.)

Then eat a portion of dark green leafy vegetables as they contain the most usable calcium. I have found the extracted juice from barley grass to be the most nutritious and it contains more calcium than other vegetables. You can grow your own and juice it if you like but I prefer using the dried juice in powder form as it is more convenient, especially when I travel.

And in case you are still nervous about this calcium issue here is information to reassure you:

In a study conducted for more than twelve years on 77,761 women between the ages of thirty-four to fifty-nine years, it was found that, "There was no evidence that higher intakes of milk or dietary calcium reduced fracture risk. There was no significant difference in the risk of hip fracture between women who drank two or more glasses of milk per day and women who drank one or less per week" (*American Journal of Public Health*, 1997).

Previous research shows that too much salt can cause loss of calcium as can gluten, the protein found in the grain portion (not the leaves) of wheat, oats, rye, and barley. I have found osteoporosis is often a symptom of gluten intolerance and it is best to avoid these foods. You can still eat a variety of carbohydrates that are gluten-free such as potatoes, corn, millet, quinoa, yams, and rice. Smoking cigarettes and coffee and tea consumption are also known to contribute to calcium loss. Try to reduce your salt intake by using natural herb or vegetable salts and seasonings. Some of these so-called health salts are still very salty. They are white in color with a few specks of herbs; the seasonings should be full of herbs and spices. Supplementation is also not the route to go as we see from the following: a nineteen-member panel prepared the latest information on dietary recommendations and after looking at more than 5000 studies, "strongly condemned the use of dietary supplements, maintaining that there was no convincing evidence that calcium supplements were necessary to prevent osteoporosis" (*South African Medical Journal* 3). In plain English, taking calcium or other mineral supplements has been shown to be of little or no value, so stop wasting your money! Besides, you can only use (if you have an efficient system) 4–10 percent of the available nutrients in these supplements due to their inorganic structure. Usable calcium has to go through the photosynthesis process that only plants go through; that is one of the reasons that plant food is such a reliable source of calcium and other nutrients. Read what the *Journal of International Medicine* had to say about the causes of osteoporosis:

Osteoporosis constitutes an important health problem in modern Western countries and is an increasing problem in the Far East. The clinical condition has no one basis, but many different factors have been suggested to contribute to its development, such as low peak bone mass, early menopause, sedentary lifestyle, cigarette smoking, slender figure, and various dietary components, such as daily calcium intake. The mean dietary consumption of calcium varies throughout the world from 150–200 mg per day in the Far East to 500–600 mg per day in the United States to 1000–1200 mg per day in the Nordic countries. The dissimilar intake of calcium in the different countries with the same incidence of osteoporotic fractures points to the fact that osteoporosis is a multifacto-

rial disease, where calcium is one of the important contributing factors
(*Journal of Internal Medicine* 161–168).

The article goes on to say that sunlight (for the manufacture of vitamin D), hormones such as parathyroid hormone, growth hormone,
estrogen, and progesterone enhance the absorption of calcium, while
glucocorticoids, excess thyroid hormone, and possibly calcitonin suppress the absorption of calcium.

Remember that to manufacture sufficient vitamin D, unheated, unprocessed, unsaturated fats are required in the diet.

The article in the *Journal of Internal Medicine* quoted above continues, "Instead of focusing on the exact number of milligrams of calcium
that should be included in the diet, one should rather center upon making sufficient efforts to maximize utilization of that calcium."

Other factors affecting calcium balance are certain supplements. Vitamin C in supplement form is consumed in large amounts, resulting in the
formation of oxalates, which reduce the bioavailability of calcium. Considering that our recommended daily intake of vitamin C is only about
60–150 mg, it is easy to take an excess in supplement form, as most supplements are from 500–1000 mg and are often taken one to three times
daily. Dietary fiber consumed in large amounts (as when adding bran to
meals) interferes with calcium absorption as do zinc, vitamin A, and iron
supplementation. Reason enough, yet again, not to take supplements.

Caffeine and alcohol increase the urinary excretion of calcium. Irra-
tional mega-doses of vitamins and minerals appear to have an adverse
effect on bone status. Seems like you would be doing some serious
damage if you continue to take supplements; remember that 90–96
percent of your hard-earned cash is being flushed away along with
your bone mass.

A diet high in protein will also increase the urinary excretion of calcium. In March 1983, the *Journal of Clinical Nutrition* reported the results of the largest study ever conducted on osteoporosis. Researchers
at Michigan State University and other major universities found that by
age sixty-five in the U.S.:

- Male vegetarians had an average bone loss of 3 percent; women 18
  percent
- Male meat eaters had an average bone loss of 7 percent; women 35
  percent

By the time a woman reaches the age of sixty-five, the average meat-eating woman in the U.S. has lost more than one third of her skeletal structure. In contrast, vegetarian women tend to remain more active, maintain erect postures, and are less likely to fracture or break bones, even with their increased physical activity. If their bones do break or fracture, they heal faster and more completely. So there you have it: if you want strong bones as you age, follow a vegetarian diet.

Where Do Hormones Fit in Here?

The endocrine system is intricately involved in maintaining bone density and blood calcium levels. To isolate one hormone (estrogen) out of dozens and one gland (the ovaries) out of several is ridiculous and dangerous. No *one* gland or hormone works on its own. The endocrine system is like a large orchestra, conducted by the pituitary gland; if one member of the orchestra is not present or not doing its job the whole company suffers.

The usual approach is to encourage women to take Hormone Replacement Therapy (HRT) in the form of estrogen. I have personally dealt with many women who have developed breast cancer after being on HRT, which resulted in radical mastectomies. HRT is not the wonder cure it is made out to be. Many women have found that their bone density is worse after being on HRT. A huge study observing more than one million women, conducted in the U.K. by Cancer Research U.K., National Health Services, and the Medical Research Council, indicated that chances of breast cancer are increased by 50 percent when on HRT.

Rather, we should be looking at the whole body, including the entire endocrine system, and following a lifestyle that encourages overall health. The Perfect Health program, starting with the five steps, will do this.

Osteoporosis can be reversed and we have seen that when the above guidelines are followed, there is marked improvement in bone density. Usually within a year, a noticeable difference can be seen.

RECAP

To obtain the right calcium and follow a lifestyle that promotes bone density and strong teeth you need:

- Sunlight—twenty to thirty minutes a day is needed to convert cholesterol into vitamin D, which is needed to use calcium. Without vitamin D you cannot utilize calcium
- Exercise—a minimum of twenty to thirty minutes a day with regular weight-bearing exercise
- The right fats—essential fatty acids and polyunsaturated fats from raw plant sources are essential for the hormonal system to work correctly. These need to be taken on a daily basis and taking flaxseed oil or a balanced blend that contains flaxseed oil (one to three tablespoons) would be ideal
- Low animal protein diet (see chapter seven)
- A high plant-based diet—at least 75 percent raw alkaline-forming fruit and vegetables

Just the first three of the Perfect Health five steps will get you there:

1. Try to eat one meal each day that is just fruit.
2. Eat fresh or dried fruit and vegetables in between meals if you crave sweet or savory foods.
3. Start all cooked meals with raw vegetables.

You also need to cut down on or remove:

- Caffeine
- Salt
- Gluten (wheat, oats, rye, and barley—if gluten intolerance is suspected, remember there is no gluten in the sprouted leaves of grains such as barley)
- Processed food such as refined sugar and flour
- Any substance that upsets the endocrine system and that could indirectly cause osteoporosis. Sugar, alcohol, caffeine, artificial sweeteners and heated fats are just a few examples
- Dietary supplements should be avoided (remember that good

old vitamin C in supplement form can contribute to osteo-porosis and that is the safest supplement to take!). The right nutrients should come directly from your diet and any extra nutrients from freshly extracted or dried vegetable juices, es-pecially barley grass juice

CHAPTER SEVEN

Protein and Meat
Is There a Difference?

MOST PEOPLE THINK that protein and meat are one and the same, and that without any animal flesh in your diet you will not get enough protein. In fact, in all the years of dealing with diet the greatest fear most people have is not taking in enough protein. I would go as far to say that many people fear lack of protein more than they do death. This just goes to show what a good job the meat industry has done in marketing its products. Before we examine these misconceptions, let's first find out what protein is, why we need it, and how much we need.

Protein is made up of twenty-three (some textbooks say twenty-two) amino acids, eight of which our adult bodies cannot manufacture and that they need to obtain from our diet (babies need a ninth and some say a tenth amino acid, which are found in breast milk). Amino acids are the building blocks of protein. They form the different types of protein our bodies need, of which there are many thousands.

Originally it was taught that our bodies need to take in the eight essential amino acids at each meal. But in recent years it has been found that we have an *amino acid pool* from which our body draws or into which it deposits amino acids as it needs them. This amino acid pool is in the blood, the liver, and the cells. If you eat too much of one type of amino acid it is deposited in the amino acid pool. Then when there is too little of any of the amino acids in the food you eat, the body withdraws what it needs from the amino acid pool. You can begin to understand where the idea of bacon and eggs for breakfast, cheese for lunch, and meat for dinner originated, especially considering that it was thought that animal products were our only reliable source of protein. We now know that even on a fruit diet adequate amounts of protein can be supplied to the body (refer to the charts at the back of the book).

This gets me back to how much protein is needed. In his book *Nature of Protein Requirements*, N. S. Scrimshaw is of the opinion that the average young man leading a fairly active life needs just thirty grams (about one ounce) of protein per day. This is far lower than the generally accepted norm. Guyton's *Textbook of Medical Physiology* (seventh edition) states that the body loses about twenty to thirty grams of protein per day, "therefore to prevent a net loss of protein from the body one must ingest a minimum of twenty to thirty grams of protein each day," although "…to be on the safe side, sixty to seventy-five grams (two ounces) is recommended" (833).

An easy way to work out your protein needs is to make sure you get 0.035 ounces (one gram) of protein for every 4½ pounds (two kilograms) of body weight.

We mainly need protein for growth and repair, and the period that we grow the fastest is during the first six months of our lives. During this time nature has provided us with the most perfect food: breast milk. The average percentage of protein in this milk is a mere 1.6 percent—just a little more than the average fruit! As adults we need protein only for repair (especially as we often have damaging habits such as smoking and drinking). But the average adult in Western society consumes far more than is needed, resulting in calcium being lost from the body through the urine. (Remember that calcium is used to neutralize the acidity caused from too much protein in the diet.) The danger in this society, therefore, is not that we don't get enough protein, but ensuring that we don't get too much. Surprisingly enough, all fruits and vegetables contain protein, with many of them, such as bananas, tomatoes, carrots, avocados, and nuts, containing all eight essential amino acids. The protein content in these foods is:

- 1 medium banana—0.035 ounces (1 g)
- 1 medium tomato—0.07 ounces (2 g)
- 1 medium carrot—0.035 ounces (1 g)
- 1 small avocado—0.07 (2 g)
- 1 cup almonds—just less than one ounce (20–25 g)
- 1 cup cashews—0.5 ounces (15.3 g)

Remember that protein levels differ from crop to crop and within each variety so this is a general guideline. (For additional information on the nutritional content of fruits and vegetables, see the tables at the back of the book.)

The China Study shows that "consumption of a lot of protein, especially animal protein, is also linked to chronic disease. Americans consume one third more protein than do Chinese and 70 percent of American protein comes from animals, while only 7 percent of Chinese protein does. Those Chinese who eat the most protein and especially the most animal protein also have the highest rates of 'diseases of affluence,' like heart disease, cancer, and diabetes" (*The New York Times*, 1991). According to the research, when animal protein is ingested, cholesterol is ingested with it. All animal products contain cholesterol including so-called low-fat dairy products, fish, and chicken. I mention this here as many people are of the opinion that only eggs and red meat contain cholesterol. No fruit or vegetable, however, has the ability to manufacture cholesterol as animals do. You need a liver to make cholesterol. Therefore no plant food, including nuts and avocado, contains cholesterol, as no plant has a liver. In fact, we now know that eating avocados and raw, unsalted nuts on a regular basis actually helps to lower cholesterol levels!

The research conducted by Dr. Campbell also shows that those who consume the most protein and have the highest cholesterol levels are not only prone to the "diseases of affluence" but also show a tendency to get cancer of the colon. Dr. Campbell concludes that, "We're basically a vegetarian species and should be consuming a wide variety of plant foods and minimizing our intake of animal foods." It is clear from Dr. Campbell's research that man is a lot healthier if he consumes very little or no animal products. Dr. Campbell, who grew up in a farming community and was a big meat eater, changed his diet radically to exclude all animal products as a result of this research. Talk about convincing evidence!

Quoting from another one of my favorite authorities on the subject, Professor Meyer, in his book *Fruit for Thought*, "By consuming adequate quantities of fruit, a subject can supply his total protein requirements." And "considering all aspects; a fruitarian diet can easily supply the protein requirements of the human body, as well as the energy requirements, provided that it contains suitable quantities of avocado and/or nuts" (48).

It makes a lot of sense to stick to a high fruit and vegetable diet, especially considering the antibiotics and hormones that are fed to animals. These ensure that they grow quicker so that the farmers can realize a speedy profit. It is now thought that this hormone-laden meat could be responsible for our children maturing at a much younger age than those of earlier generations. (With earlier maturation comes earlier degeneration.) It is also thought that many of the hormones used to promote growth are estrogen-based, contributing to estrogen overload, which can not only contribute to cancer but also breast formation in men. Then there is sodium sulfite, a chemical substance that is used on red meat to retain its natural color. Research shows us that this substance could aggravate or even trigger asthma attacks, anaphylactic shock, and other respiratory tract problems. In processed meats such as baloney, polony, and Vienna or hotdog sausages (which, by the way, are made of the leftover snouts, udders, lips, eyes, and ears), sodium nitrate and nitrite are used as colorants and preservatives. The question here, according to food scientists Erik Millstone and John Abraham in their book, *Additives: A Guide for Everyone*, "is not whether nitrate consumption can contribute to cancer, but how much cancer is being caused" (87). Under the circumstances, it seems that animal proteins are not such a wise choice.

If you still enjoy eating meat, then as a rule, fish is best, then organic free-range chickens, then venison (no hormones or antibiotics), and then organic red meat that has not been treated with sodium sulfite. Ask your butcher for untreated organic meat. And this brings us to Step 5.

STEP 5: Try to Eat Animal Protein No More Than Once a Day, Preferably No More Than Three Times a Week

Try not to eat animal protein more than once a day; in other words if you have had some fish for lunch, don't eat more protein such as chicken or lamb for dinner. Have a properly combined starch meal instead. Even better, try to eat animal protein not more than every other day.

If you are a vegetarian or if you plan to become one, then you should try and include at least a quarter to half a cup of raw, unsalted nuts every day. Remember that groundnuts are classed as legumes rather than nuts. Legumes are difficult to digest as they are generally cooked. Cooked protein is more difficult to digest and can contain trisaccharides or glucose molecules that are linked in chains and are difficult to digest. Soaking legumes overnight in filtered water before cooking makes them more digestible. Processed soy products that are made to look like minced beef or other meat products are not generally the most nutritious of the legumes to eat due to the intense processing they go through to make them look and taste like meat. In fact, I have found it best to minimize soy. When eating nuts, remember to eat and combine them as a protein, for example, with neutral vegetables and not starches, although they can be combined with acid and sub-acid fruit. Some nuts such as pecans and Brazil nuts are low in protein and can be eaten with other fruit and occasionally with starches. For example, you may be quite comfortable eating pecans in a salad followed by a pasta dish.

It is clear that you do not have to eat animal flesh or products to receive your daily protein requirements. Nor do you have to eat a complete protein at each meal, if you are on a properly combined, high-raw diet. If, however, you enjoy meat, fish, and poultry, try not to eat these more than once a day, keeping your intake of red meat down to a maximum of three times per week. And remember that in the society in which we live, there is more chance of getting too much protein, with resultant kidney damage, loss of calcium, and degenerative disease, than there is of getting too little!

There are some people who feel better when they include animal protein in their diets on a regular basis; this may be for psychological reasons (fear of weakness, lack of understanding) or for physiological reasons. These physiological reasons may be due to a digestive tract that does not secrete enough hydrochloric acid to activate the intrinsic factor that helps us absorb and use vitamin B12. This could result in a B12 deficiency, which you may believe can be corrected by eating meat. Statistics show that on average 40 percent of vegetarians *and* meat eaters suffer from a vitamin B12 deficiency, indicating that lack of animal flesh is clearly not the cause.

There are so many reasons for B12 deficiencies but many people now believe that being too clean—in other words sterilizing everything possible—will destroy many of the friendly bacteria that make B12. So using antiseptic soaps and bleaching agents on everything can, in fact, upset the delicate balance of friendly bacteria and this can result in serious health problems. You can be clean without sterilizing every surface; you will be cleaner if the good bacteria are allowed to control the bad bacteria. Some people also believe that chlorine in our drinking water sterilizes not only the water but our digestive tracts and this contributes to a B12 problem (one of the many reasons to filter your water). We do know that a B12 deficiency in rural communities is extremely rare and uncommon in both meat eaters and vegetarians but more common in Westernized, more affluent communities. Whether this is due to over-sterilization from our water treatments or household cleaning materials, stress, consumption of other processed foods, or all of the above is unclear. I suggest taking regular blood tests (every few years or so) and checking your B12 levels as well as other nutrients just to make sure you are on track and to give you peace of mind. The issue to focus on is not whether you are a vegetarian but to make sure you are eating a form of protein on a daily basis that you are comfortable with, and that your digestive tract is healthy so that you can absorb the nutrients you need for vibrant health.

Recent diet books have indicated that people who have type-O blood need to eat meat to be healthy. This is like saying that blue-eyed people should be vegetarian, or that dark-skinned people should eat meat. What I have found in many people who are type-O, including my husband Mark, is that when they eat animal protein it causes high blood pressure and extra weight, and when they discontinue eating animal flesh their weight drops as does their blood pressure. Only people living a wealthy Westernized lifestyle can afford the luxury of blood group diets and at the end of the day people benefit from these diets because they are instructed to remove all processed foods and gluten and, no matter what your blood group, your health would improve if you did this. At the end of the day it is a physiological fact that we need protein, but that we need very little. We know that animal protein is the most expensive protein for us to eat in that it has the worst side effects for our health. The less we eat it, the better, no matter what blood group we are. There is little independent research to back up this claim and I have known many type-O vegetarians who have excellent health, including some of my children and my husband!

At the end of the day, you live in your body and only you know what is comfortable and right for you. Some people have nut allergies and if so there are a variety of options. Sesame seed paste (tahini) is a very concentrated source of protein containing as much as chicken and fish (20–25 percent) and pumpkin seeds contain even more protein.

The digestive tract is controlled by the endocrine system and many things such as caffeine, alcohol, gluten intolerance, stress, cigarettes, contraceptive pills, artificial sweeteners, etc., can upset this system and this could result in digestive disorders or malfunction. A common problem is leaky gut, a syndrome caused by you not digesting proteins properly. (See chapter four.) This is the main reason why proper food-combining alleviates so many allergies.

Below is research to support eating less animal protein:

- "Red meat, especially hamburgers, is associated with an increase in non-Hodgkin's Lymphoma" (*Journal of the American Medical Association*, May 1996)
- A "high intake of animal protein—more than 95 gm per day—showed a significantly higher risk of osteoporosis. Plant protein showed the least. (The average person following a Westernized diet can easily consume 120 grams of protein daily)" (*American Journal of Epidemiology*, March 1996)
- "The latest on protein levels—45 gm is required daily for women and 55 gm daily for men. The average intake in the U.K. and U.S.A. is easily 80–90 gm daily" (*South African Medical Journal*, Dr. Walker)
- "A diet high in fat and meat increases cancer" (*Cancer Epidemiology*, January 1996)
- "People consuming more meat spend more money on medical expenses and cost the government more in medical costs" (*Preventative Medicine*, November 1995)
- "High intakes of meat and red meat were associated with a significant increase in breast cancer" (*International Journal of Cancer*, January 1996)
- "Increased intake of animal fat and animal protein shows a corresponding increase in breast cancer" (*Asia Pacific Journal Public Health*, 1994)
- *The Lancet* (October 1991) published research that clearly states that the only way to get rid of arthritis is a vegetarian, plant-based diet
- Tests on rats, eating a 20 percent protein diet, all developed cancer, but those on a 5 percent protein diet were cancer-free. On a low-fat, high-protein diet, the rats developed hardening of the arteries and very high cholesterol levels, and after one year, 75 percent had developed kidney disease (*Health Revolution*, 1989)
- "In the digestion of protein we are constantly exposed to large

amounts of ammonia in our intestinal tract" (Dr. Willard Visek, Clinical Sciences, University of Illinois Medical School)

- Ammonia behaves like a carcinogen, meaning it kills cells, increases infections, affects the rate at which cells divide, and increases the mass of the lining of intestines. Statistics show that in the colon, cancer parallels the concentration of ammonia. Ammonia is also formed when we badly combine foods. This clearly shows why cancer of the digestive tract is the most common form of cancer

- "Compared to carbohydrates, the digestion of protein requires seven times the amount of water to flush out the ammonia produced" (Dr. Nathan Smith, Professor of Sports Medicine, University of Washington)

- "A potent carcinogen, Malonaldehyde (a chemical that begins to form in flesh soon after death), has been identified in beef and smaller amounts in pork, chicken, and fish" (Dr. Raymond Shamberger, Cleveland Clinic Foundation)

In 1968, when Danish researchers tested muscle energy levels of men cyclists, they found the following:

- Those eating a meat, milk, and egg diet cycled for 57 minutes before muscle failure
- Those eating a meat and vegetable diet cycled for 114 minutes before muscle failure
- Those on a vegetable, grain, and fruit diet cycled for 167 minutes before muscle failure

Yes, you can lose weight on any diet including high-protein diets, but your health will deteriorate. I have yet to find someone on these diets who does not develop some health problem somewhere down the line.

It is a physiological fact that the human body needs a high alkaline-forming diet to maintain health. This will only work on an 80 percent raw fruit and vegetable diet. A high alkaline-forming diet promotes a healthy immune system and only in the right alkaline environment will fuel be converted into energy efficiently. A 75–80 percent alkaline-forming, plant-based diet will do this. If fuel cannot be converted into energy it will be stored and weight problems will result. If you follow the five Perfect Health steps, you will easily have an 80 percent alkaline-forming diet.

Heart Association Warns of Risk in High-Protein Diets

"Despite their popularity, high-protein diets aren't making good on their promise of long-term weight loss," says a new scientific advisory from the American Heart Association. Moreover, the AHA says the diets are a health risk for people who stay on them beyond short periods of time. "In general, quick weight-loss diets don't work for most people," says Robert H. Eckel, M.D., co-author of a scientific advisory from the AHA's nutrition committee. "It's important for the public to understand that no scientific evidence supports the claim that these diets work," Dr. Eckel says.

"Some of the diets increase fat intake and reduce nutritionally rich foods such as fruits and vegetables, which is not a good approach to meeting a person's long-term dietary needs," says Dr. Eckel. "Many of these diets fail to provide essential vitamins, minerals, fiber, and other nutritional elements, in addition to their high-fat content." Eating large amounts of high-fat animal foods over a sustained period has been shown to increase the risk of coronary heart disease, diabetes, stroke, and several types of cancer, the advisory says.

If you feel you need more detailed information on the protein issues you can get hold of our Natural Health and Nutrition Course from www.mary-anns.com, or read *The China Study* by Dr. Colin Campbell, *Dr. Dean Ornish's Program for Reversing Heart Disease* by Dr. Dean Ornish, or *The Food Revolution* by John Robbins.

RECAP

- These five Perfect Health steps will help you find the right balance and ensure you are receiving all the vitamins, minerals, proteins, carbohydrates, and fats that you need, while keeping the important alkaline balance. Start with at least one of them today as you keep reading and make small adjustments rather than one huge change:

1. Eat at least one fruit meal per day.
2. All snacks should be fresh or dried fruit or vegetables.

3. Start all cooked food with some raw vegetables.
4. Try not to eat a concentrated protein with a concentrated starch at the same meal.
5. Try to eat no more than one animal protein meal a day.

- Using these steps you should find yourself eating one meal a day that consists entirely of fresh fruit and nuts, a second meal that includes fresh raw and cooked vegetables with a natural unprocessed starch such as potatoes, brown rice, corn, sweet potatoes, or yams, and a third meal of raw and cooked vegetables with one kind of protein if you feel the need for extra protein besides the nuts. If you are a very active athlete you may have a second meal including more carbohydrates or starches as mentioned, or a second fruit meal

- If you are an inactive person who battles with your weight, make sure you eat starches no more than once a day, with the third meal being just raw and/or cooked neutral vegetables

CHAPTER EIGHT

The High-Fat, Low-Fat, No-Fat Diet
Fats: Are They Needed and What about Cholesterol?

OF ALL THE NUTRIENTS we desperately need on a daily basis, none have been as maligned as fat! We have come through the era of no-fat and low-fat everything; milk to salad dressings to chocolates to candy have been manipulated to remove or lower the fat content. In fact, at some point all our health problems were supposedly because of fat in our diets.

Well, some lowered their fat intake and many removed it completely and what have we found? Since 1995 obesity has increased by 100 million people, cancer and diabetes is on the rise, and there are more auto-immune diseases than ever before. Now almost everyone I speak to has a disease or condition related to the hormonal system.

The problem is we desperately need fats! If we do not take in enough of these essential fats we will continually find ourselves craving savory foods. The craving for cheese, fries, burgers, hotdogs, and other fried foods clearly indicates that you lack essential fatty acids. And if we do not take in the right essential fats on a daily basis almost any and everything can go wrong, from blood pressure to blood sugar, allergies, hay fever, arthritis, gout, fibromyalgia, constipation, sleep problems, low muscle tone, and skin, kidney, liver, lung, and heart problems. You name it, it will relate back to the hormonal system and this system simply will not work properly without the two essential fats commonly known as Omega 3 and Omega 6.

Yes, fats are essential in your diet, but the majority of people consume the wrong kinds of fats.

First, fat is needed as a source of heat and energy for the body. Our body temperature needs to be consistent, no matter what the weather, and we need energy at the most basic level just to keep our hearts beating. Second, fat is also needed for padding and insulating the organs and nerves. I'll never forget how uncomfortable it was to sit after the first fourteen-day fast I completed—I simply had insufficient padding and found it more comfortable to stand until my fat reserves had been rebuilt. Next, fats play an essential role in the diet; they are needed to help with the absorption of the fat-soluble vitamins A, D, E, and K. I find it interesting that all fruits (see tables in the back) and vegetables contain vitamin A (actually beta-carotene, which is the precursor to vitamin A), which is a fat-soluble vitamin, along with fat—nature has made sure that the vitamin A is absorbable and assimilated because of the presence of fat. Also, fats are a source of essential fatty acids. These are needed for the proper functioning of the endocrine system that controls hormone production, growth, reproductive activity, production of vitamin B12 in the intestines, and for helping to make calcium and phosphorus more available. Lack of, or insufficient, fatty acids can result in any of the problems mentioned above and more problems such as gallstones, loss of hair, impaired growth and reproductive functioning, and kidney, prostate, and menstrual disturbances.

As previously mentioned, there are two essential fats we need on a daily basis. The first one is known as linoleic acid (known as LA or Omega 6) and alpha-linolenic acid (known as ALA or Omega 3).

Contrary to some information, Omega 3 and 6 can only be obtained from plant sources as only plants have the ability to insert a double bond at the carbon atom numbers 3 and 6. Omega 6 is found abundantly in a variety of plants and the oils extracted from these plants, such as sunflower, corn, and sesame seeds along with the cold-pressed oils from these plants. Omega 6 is found in almost every fruit and vegetable, including avocados, nuts, and seeds. It is very difficult to develop a deficiency of Omega 6 on a natural diet; however, if you eat very little or no natural fats and only consume low-fat commercial foods, it could easily develop. Symptoms of a deficiency of this essential fat are eczema-like skin eruptions, loss of hair, liver and/or kidney degeneration, excessive sweating accompanied by thirst, drying up of glands, susceptibility to infections, failure to heal wounds (indicating a run-down immune system), sterility in males, miscarriage, arthritis, and related conditions such as gout or fibromyalgia, heart and circulatory problems, and growth retardation. These symptoms can all be reversed by adding natural plants foods that contain fats.

The second essential fatty acid is Omega 3 or alpha-linolenic acid, which is possibly more important than Omega 6 as it is much easier to develop a deficiency in it. Most people consume too much Omega 6 and not enough Omega 3. Both essential fats are found in most plant food but Omega 3 is extremely concentrated in cold-pressed organically grown flaxseed oil (also known as linseed but not the commercial types used in treating wood, which are toxic) and also found freely in dark green leafy vegetables.

Omega 3 deficiency symptoms are growth retardation, weakness, impairment of vision and learning ability, motor incoordination, tingling sensations in arms and legs, behavioral changes, high triglycerides, high blood pressure, sticky platelets, tissue inflammation, water retention, dry skin, mental deterioration, low metabolic rate (causing weight and digestive problems), and immune dysfunction. Can you imagine how many people are on medication for high blood pressure, arthritis, or heart disease who could just sort it out by obtaining this essential fat through their diets? Including a good source of flaxseed oil in your diet on a daily basis can go a long way toward correcting these symptoms. I suggest you start with one to three tablespoons daily for the first six to twelve months or at least until your symptoms clear and then reduce this to one to two teaspoons daily as a maintenance amount. More importantly, listen to your body; you may find you need to continue with a higher intake or that you need to decrease your intake sooner, especially if you have no other fats in your diet. If your symptoms return after being on pure flax for some time it may indicate that you are overloading your body with Omega 3, so discontinue the pure flaxseed oil for a week and then start taking a flaxseed blend, ensuring you are including other natural fats in your diet. For more information on which product we use go to www.mary-anns.com.

A lot of nonsense has been thrown about concerning Omega 3, with a lot of companies promoting a variety of EFA (essential fatty acids) or Omega 3 products. Fish oil, in particular, is promoted in some circles as the miracle cure to every known health problem. The claim made is that fish oil is loaded with Omega 3, EPA (eicosapentaenoic acid), and DHA (docosahexanoic acid). So to help you sort out the facts from the fiction, I will explain what the truth is regarding these fats.

Omega 3 is an essential fat and as explained above can be made only by plants. It is then converted in humans into five Omega 3 derivatives—two of them are DHA and EPA. Just like the other derivatives, these two are essential and necessary, but you do not need to take them as your body will produce them as much as is needed (much like your body converts beta-carotene into vitamin A at the rate you need it). Think of derivatives as children, grandchildren, great-grandchildren, etc. EPA is the great-grandchild of Omega 3 and DHA the great, great, great-grandchild. So as much as they are part of the family of Omega 3 they are not actually Omega 3. The companies that promote fish oil will tell you that it is the best source of Omega 3, which is not the truth as you are only getting two family members (derivatives) and not the original parent Omega 3, which is what we are designed to have.

Fish oil supplements are made by extracting the oil through a process of heat and chemical solvents; this process can result in carcinogenic by-products that are not ideal. The oils are then encapsulated with heat and you then have no way of knowing whether these oils are rancid because you cannot taste them, although you may find yourself tasting fish for hours afterward, indicating clearly that the oil is not digestible and is indeed rancid. Fish oil also comes loaded with cholesterol. If you overdose on these supplements they can cause serious immune problems. EPA and DHA are needed by the body along with vitamin E to be efficiently processed. Fish oil lacks vitamin E whereas flaxseed oil and other cold-pressed vegetable oils have an abundance of vitamin E. Eating fats from plants allows your body to make all the EPA and DHA it needs, whereas you could be seriously overdosing when taking fish oil. It seems somewhat insane to be killing fish to extract the oils when you can get everything you need from plant foods in a far better, more natural and usable state. Some people claim that we do not have the ability to convert Omega 3 to EPA and DHA. This is utter nonsense; the only reason we cannot convert Omega 3 is because we are not getting it in our diet in the first place. If you happen to be one of the less than 2 percent of people who are genetically unable to do this conversion, then eat fresh fish instead. The fat is only heated once when you cook it and does not contain chemical solvents, although you may be getting a good dose of heavy metals like mercury. Then make sure you daily drink a tall glass of barley grass juice as the chlorophyll will help to neutralize these heavy metals.

Cholesterol is produced only in animals, so all animal products (not just eggs) contain a certain amount of cholesterol. Anything that has a liver makes cholesterol, including fish, and there is no plant in the world that has a liver. But according to Dr. Henry Bieler in his book *Food Is Your Best Medicine,* the real problem with fats is not so much the cholesterol content, but whether the fat has been heated. He says that overeating fats and oils, as long as they are in their natural state, cannot cause arterial disease. The body merely stores the excess as fat. It is only when we consume unnatural fats (such as tea and coffee creamers, margarine, and fried foods) or natural fats that have been altered by being overheated, that the trouble arises. Why are heated fats so bad for us? Quite simply, we do not have the enzymes that are able to break down fats heated to more than 100°C–160°C (depending on the fat). It is for this reason that frying is out of the question from a health point-of-view as fried fats are heated way over 100°C–160°C. Adding a bit of olive oil or butter (if you must) to vegetables after they have been cooked poses no threat, as the temperature at which the butter melts is way below 100°C. Included in the category of natural fats that have been heated are all the oils that have been pressed or extracted from seeds, such as sunflower, sesame, and olive oil. Unless the labels state that they have been "cold-pressed" or are "extra-virgin," all oils are heated numerous times in the extraction process. All margarines are heated during processing and even butter used in baking cakes or cookies is heated above 100°C. (Although heated butter is easier for us to use than most heated fats, with the exception of coconut oil.) Both butter and coconut oil are a saturated fat and, as such, are stable during the heating process—they do not change shape and are easier for us to digest than a heated, unsaturated fat. For this reason heated, saturated fats in small quantities occasionally can be tolerated by most people without any serious problems.

We have been led to believe by the oil and margarine advertising companies that all vegetable fats are better than any animal fats. But is this true? Let us compare the relative merits of butter and margarine. Butter is not heated during processing. You can make your own butter:

simply beat cream past the thick stage to when it separates. Then rinse the fatty part that is formed and pour off the watery part. You then have unsalted butter. If you prefer salted butter, just add a little salt. According to the dairy industry, the amount of salt in butter is about 2 percent. Occasionally annatto (a natural coloring extracted from a tree) is used. The body is capable of handling this fat quite comfortably. Whereas the same cannot be said for margarine, which is heated several times before it eventually reaches our tables.

Here is a brief summary of how oils and margarines are manufactured. This method is approved internationally, according to the oil companies. However, they neglect to mention that this approval does not necessarily mean that these products are good for you! The seeds, from which the oil is extracted, are first decorticated, or husked. They are then subjected to steam so that the cells will rupture with ease and thus release more oil. The seeds are then dried, using a heat process once again. At this stage, the seeds pass through an expeller, leaving about 20 percent of the oil in the caked seed. Hexane, a benzene derivative, is now percolated through the leftover seed-cake, in order to extract the remaining oil. The oil is then filtered and neutralized with caustic soda. Bleaching follows at this point, by using bleaching earth and by heating the oil in a vacuum. Here, the oil is winterized, or cooled to a very low temperature. This is to filter out harmless, natural wax crystals. Under the vacuum the oil is heated yet again, this time to between 220° and 290°C, to render the oil odorless. Apparently we would find the natural smell of the seeds offensive. To this insipid, odorless concoction, colorant is now added. Unless of course we prefer to buy light oil, then the paler, the better and no color is added. (As if calories had anything to do with color!) The oil is now ready for bottling to be sold to us as salad or cooking oil.

In the manufacturing of margarine, the oil goes through all the above processes and is then hydrogenated in the presence of a nickel catalyst. This is to ensure that this denatured, destroyed oil can be spread like butter. But that's not all! Whey, a watery fluid separated from milk, is now added, as are butter flavoring and the preservative sodium benzoate. This particular preservative has been found to result in fetal damage and respiratory problems such as asthma and bronchitis. Yet despite this questionable process and equally questionable product, we are constantly told that margarine is healthier for us than butter!

Let's face it, genuine old-fashioned butter and cold-pressed oils just have to be better. I'd like to add here that this should not give you license to over-indulge in cream and butter as any fat, particularly animal fat, in excess is not ideal. Most cancer associations state that too much fat in the diet can cause cancer, and although they don't state whether the research was done using heated or unheated fats, there does seem to be evidence that heated fats and animal fats are the culprit. Animal fats, it appears, can contribute to cancer due to the hormones used to encourage milk production.

When it comes to fats, the consumer is frequently baffled by the terms *saturated*, *unsaturated*, *polyunsaturated*, and *monounsaturated*. I sometimes think that these terms are thrown at us from all angles, in the hope that we will become so confused that we will believe all the advertising claims about fats and buy the latest product! I hope to be able to clear up some of this confusion.

Saturated Fats

Saturated fats are fats that are solid at room temperature. They are found mostly in animal products such as meat, chicken, eggs, cheese, milk, and butter. **Saturated** fats are also present in coconuts. Saturated simply means that these fats do not have the ability to bond in the body as they have no open bonds; in other words, they are usually empty calories that contribute to a fat buildup or weight gain in the body although small quantities of saturated fats are used by the body for certain chemical reactions. Saturated fats, when from an animal source, are always accompanied by cholesterol. (Remember that plants are unable to manufacture cholesterol.) Cholesterol, as we all know, contributes to heart disease when consumed on a regular basis. Although it is important to remember that cholesterol is manufactured by our bodies and serves a very useful purpose, namely to manufacture cell membranes, nerve tissue, hormones, and bile acids used to digest food. Our bodies produce the right amount of cholesterol for healthy maintenance in these areas; we do not need additional cholesterol.

By consuming a diet high in fresh, raw fruit and vegetables and following the Perfect Health principles outlined in this book, you will be able to maintain the correct cholesterol blood levels that result in optimum health.

Unsaturated Fats

Unsaturated fats are fats that, in their chemical structure, have open links. This structure enables them to combine easily with various nutrients and they are therefore put to use easily in the cells. Unsaturated fats are found mainly in all nuts, seeds, and avocados. All fruits and vegetables contain small quantities of this type of fat. Unsaturated fats are liquid at room temperature.

Polyunsaturated Fats

Polyunsaturated fats are those that have large numbers of fatty acids, which in turn have open links and are therefore also easily utilized by the cells. These are also found in all fruits, vegetables, nuts, and seeds.

Monounsaturated Fats

Monounsaturated fats are fats that have a single fatty acid with open links, and are found in all fruits and vegetables.

If you are still confused about saturated, unsaturated, polyunsaturated, and monounsaturated fats, think of fats as a vehicle; in particular a bus. If the bus that is coming along in the bloodstream has all the seats taken, it would be a saturated fat as there is no space for anything else on board. If there is only one seat available on the bus it is a mono (meaning one) unsaturated (meaning not full) fat, which means there is very little space available, and if the bus has two or more seats available then it is a poly (meaning many) unsaturated fat.

The buses with seats available (both mono- and polyunsaturated fats), known collectively as unsaturated fats, are able to pick up cholesterol in the bloodstream, where it is deposited by the liver and transported to cells where it is needed to make hormones such as progesterone, testosterone, and estrogen. Wherever you find essential fatty acids you will find the bus with one or more empty seats (mono- and polyunsaturated fats). So eating avocados, raw nuts, seeds, sweet corn on the cob, olives, dark green leafy vegetables, and cold-pressed oils will actually help you lower cholesterol levels as they pick up cholesterol and move it out of the bloodstream to the cells where it is needed. Cholesterol is also used to build membranes of new cells, for brain function, and to manufacture vitamin D in the skin when exposed to sunlight (see chapter ten). Cholesterol is essential to our bodies and good cholesterol is the kind our liver makes while the bad cholesterol is the kind we eat from animal sources. We are led to believe that LDL (low density lipoprotein) is the bad cholesterol, but we actually need it; it is just that when our diet is out of balance it increases to a level that is considered dangerous.

When the cells don't get enough cholesterol to do their job, they send a message to the liver to make more cholesterol. The liver obliges and makes more, but if the cholesterol is not being transported efficiently it collects in the bloodstream. Very often people with high cholesterol problems crave fatty foods as the body tries to get the message across that it needs essential fats to help move the cholesterol to where it is needed. These people also often have other health problems related to the endocrine system, clearly indicating that the cholesterol is not able to reach the cells where it would be used to correct endocrine (hormonal) problems. The endocrine system controls just about every function in the body, from blood pressure and blood sugar, to brain, kidney, liver, lung, bowel, and skin functions. Also appetite, metabolism, and water retention are controlled as well as allergies, hay fever, and gout. These are just a few of the functions of the endocrine system. If there are not enough essential fatty acids (EFAs) in your diet then these hormones cannot be made and without EFAs the other important unsaturated fats (unheated) don't get into the body to transport the cholesterol out of your bloodstream, where the liver dumps it, and to the cells where it is needed; this very often results in high cholesterol levels.

Studies from Loma Linda and New Mexico universities have shown that blood cholesterol levels are dramatically lowered when raw nuts are incorporated into the diet. Researchers say that it is the unsaturated fats in nuts that help lower cholesterol levels. Nuts also contain plant components with antioxidant properties, which can slow the oxidation or "rusting" of LDL (bad) cholesterol. University of Georgia research has confirmed that nuts also contain plant sterols, which have been in the news recently for their cholesterol-lowering ability. All other plant sources of fats have the same effect for the same reasons and this just confirms what I have said: good fats will lower your cholesterol levels.

The renowned heart specialist Dr. Dean Ornish in his book *Reversing Heart Disease* explains that a totally vegetarian diet, regular exercise, and dealing with emotional issues can reverse heart disease and unblock arteries within two years.

Essential fatty acids also help the body to produce prostaglandins, which are essential for managing cholesterol levels. Prostaglandins (PGs) are short-lived, hormone-like chemicals that regulate cellular activities on a moment-to-moment basis. More than thirty different PGs have been identified, with each having a different function and falling into three families or categories known as Series 1, 2, and 3.

SERIES 1

Series 1 derivative (called PGE_1) keeps blood platelets from sticking together, preventing heart attacks and strokes. It helps remove sodium and excess fluid from our bodies, helping with water retention. It improves circulation and lowers blood pressure and cholesterol. It lowers the inflammatory response, relieving arthritis, and helps insulin to work more efficiently, improves nerve function, regulates calcium, and improves T-Cell functions, thus improving immune function. It also regulates the release of arachidonic acid (AA).

SERIES 2

AA is the precursor to Series 2 prostaglandins and PGE_2, one of the members of this family, promotes clot formation, water retention, and high blood pressure. It also causes inflammation, opposes PGE_1, and is considered a bad guy. AA is freely available in all animal products and this is part of the reason why animal products promote heart disease (clotting, water retention, and HBP). All foods that contain cholesterol also contain AA, so it is important to keep these foods to a minimum and certainly not consume them more than once a day and preferably not more than three times a week or not at all.

SERIES 3

Series 3 PGs are made from eicosapentaenoic acid (EPA), a derivative of Omega 3. The most powerful effect of PG_3 is that it prevents AA from being released. This would explain why good quality flaxseed oil helps reduce inflammation, which in turn alleviates gout, arthritis, and other inflammatory conditions and can prevent degenerative cardiovascular disease, water retention, and high blood pressure. EPA is also found in fish but brings with it cholesterol and is also usually heated so is not as ideal as flaxseed oil. Vitamin E is essential for the metabolic processes of essential fats. There is none in fish but plenty in flaxseed oil; so all around, unheated, organic flaxseed oil is a better option than fish oil.

RECAP

- Fats are needed by the body, but make sure that you stick to the right kinds of fat. Fruit, vegetables, nuts, seeds, and cold-pressed oils contain the correct sorts of fat. Ensure that these foods make up the bulk of your diet by following the Perfect Health five steps. And when it comes to making healthy choices for your body, butter is better than margarine, and cold-pressed vegetable oils such as flaxseed, olive, and coconut oils are better than butter. You may want to blend some of these oils together. The coconut oil will help to make the mixture spreadable or you may just want to blend some of these natural oils with butter to start with
- Remember that without the right fat you can actually slow down your metabolism as it is controlled by the endocrine system, which cannot function efficiently without essential fats. So to lose excess fat you need to eat the right fats
- Try and eat at least one of the following six sources of fat a day, plus a flax blend and barley grass juice to make sure you are obtaining sufficient fats, which will of course help to correct cholesterol levels:

  o 1–3 avocados
  o ¼–½ cup of raw unsalted nuts or seeds
  o 5–10 olives in brine
  o 2–6 sweet corn on the cob
  o 1–3 tablespoons of cold-pressed oil blend, which must include flaxseed oil as a major ingredient
  o A plate full of dark green leafy vegetables, whole or juiced, or 2–3 teaspoons of dried barley grass juice

To sum up, you need a HIGH intake of natural unheated and un-processed plant fats, a LOW intake of unheated animal fats, and NO intake of processed fats: The HIGH, LOW, NO-FAT DIET!

CHAPTER NINE

Additives
The Invisible Enemies

ADDITIVES are the body's invisible enemies—invisible because we can't see them, and we are not even alerted to their presence as they are often not listed on food packaging. As I sit here writing, I am recovering from a "run in" with one of these additives—sulfur dioxide—and I now have hives on my face, arms, and legs. Although my reaction these days is very mild compared to when I first discovered the allergy, it is still unpleasant. I remember as a young girl getting a strange rash on my face, arms, and legs and being diagnosed with sun sensitivity; I was told to stay out of the sun and given large doses of vitamin A. No one ever asked me what I had eaten and there was definitely no talk of additives. I was at a boarding school at the time and my mother would load us up with dried fruit (thinking it was a healthier option than candy), which I loved. Little did any of us realize that the preservative added to the dried fruit was the cause of my skin problem. I now always ask about additives at farm stalls when there is no label on dried fruit or if it is sold by weight and yet even with assurances that there are no preservatives, I sometimes find I have eaten dried fruit that is preserved. That is the problem: it is invisible.

I feel very strongly about being given a choice—if we choose to consume or not to consume foods containing certain additives, the decision should rest with us. But we should at least have the right to know exactly what we are eating so that we can be in a position to choose intelligently and correctly. Fortunately in the last few years labeling has become important and manufacturers are bound by law to list all the ingredients in their foods.

Listing ingredients does not automatically mean the product is good, but it does give you, the consumer, the right of first refusal.

Additives seem to adversely affect so many people, especially children. It seems that food manufacturers want to titillate our children's taste buds with flavorants, attract their eyes with colorants, and preserve their food so that it never decays, resulting in little returns to the stores. Our children are exposed to these substances in hotdogs, burgers, fries (any fast food), mayonnaise, salad dressings, soda, candy, breakfast cereals, and in fact most of the food manufactured and manmade. The easiest thing for a mother to do is stick to natural foods, read labels, and go for homemade.

Food additives refer to chemicals added deliberately during industrial food processing. The manufacturers believe that using these chemicals enhances their product and makes it easier to sell. Some of them even try and convince us that preservatives make the products safer for us. Additives are sometimes identified by the letter E, which is followed by a number. The letter E is the standard identification code in Europe for additives and there are currently more than 4,000 additives in use internationally (some books list 12,000!). It is a good idea to keep an additive book handy. Although the amounts of additives used by manufacturers are technically legal, the accumulative and combined effect of these substances can cause a tremendous amount of unnecessary pain and suffering.

Time and time again I have come across a man or woman suffering from recurring and severe migraines. This person is usually at his or her wits' end as he or she has been for every sort of test imaginable, including brain scans. After taking a look at this person's diet, I found, without exception, that one of the following additives was the cause of the trouble: caffeine, monosodium glutamate (MSG), or the artificial sweetener aspartame. In other cases where recurring bronchitis is the problem, when the additive sulfur dioxide benzoate is removed from the diet, the bronchitis miraculously disappears. You may, in fact, be following a relatively healthy diet but suffering from an irritating or even debilitating illness that could be sorted out just by removing certain additives.

For additives to be used, they must be approved and most countries are comfortable with the American Food and Drug association (FDA) approval. In other words, if the FDA approves it, it must be okay. The problem is that many of these additives are not properly tested or are tested on rats, not humans. Very seldom is any possible interaction between additives tested, either. The following from John Abraham and Eric Millstone's book, *Additives*, sums up the real issue: "As far as consumers are concerned, the crucial question is: who is getting the benefit of the doubt? If experts, officials, and government are giving the benefit to consumers then they will assume that a chemical is toxic until it is proved to be safe, but if they are giving the benefit of the doubt to industry then they will assume it to be safe until proved harmful. We believe that the benefit of the doubt has consistently been awarded to industry and not to consumers where it rightly belongs" (18).

Here follows a more detailed description of the most widely used additives, where they are found, and what possible side effects they may have. There are thousands of additives and many of them may be harmless. These are listed as they are the most commonly used and the most likely to cause health problems.

The Colorants

TARTRAZINE (E 102)

Tartrazine is a bright yellow coal tar dye, commonly found in many sweets with colors ranging from cream to yellow to orange to green. Tartrazine is generally recognized to be responsible for a wide range of allergic and intolerant symptoms, including hyperactivity in children, asthma, migraine headaches, and skin rashes. According to some research, Tartrazine is also suspected as a possible cause of cancer. Its use is prohibited in Norway and Finland and restricted in Sweden. We often make the mistake of thinking that if a food is Tartrazine-free it is safe to consume, regardless of what other additives it may contain. So even if the package proclaims it is tartrazine-free, check what other ingredients it may contain, as many of the other approved colorants can also be harmful.

ANNATO (E 160 [B])

This is a natural yellow coloring extracted from the Annato tree and used to color cheese and butter. The dairy industry may claim that it is harmless, but there is evidence that it can provoke symptoms of intolerance in people who are susceptible to urticaria (hives) or angioneurotic edema (a severe condition of hives or a bad skin rash).

ALUMINUM (E 173)

Used as a silver colorant, aluminum is also found in Ceylon (black) and green tea (though not herbal teas). Aluminum pots can oxidize and contaminate the food during the cooking process and can then be absorbed into the body. There is evidence that this metal plays a part in the onset of Alzheimer's disease or senility.

The Preservatives

SODIUM BENZOATE AND OTHER BENZOATES (E 210–E 219)

Sodium benzoate is used in all margarines and in some dried fruits, sodas, juices, and bottled sauces and salad dressings. In all related studies, levels of consumption have been found that provoke ill-health including (in some cases) fetal damage, hyperactivity, asthma, and urticaria.

SULFUR DIOXIDE AND THE SULFITING AGENTS (E 220–E 227 [INCLUDING SODIUM SULFITE])

These substances are commonly found in all dried fruit other than dark dried fruit such as dates, raisins, and prunes. If the dried fruit retains its original color, for example if the dried peaches are bright yellow and soft, then more often than not they have been treated with sulfur dioxide. It is also one of the most widely used preservatives as it is readily available and inexpensive. It is found in beer, wine, sausage meat, soups, sauces, juices, sodas, salad dressings, and dried vegetables. Sodium sulfite is used on red meat to retain the red, fresh appearance. Sulfur dioxide and sodium sulfite can reduce levels of calcium as well as enhance the carcinogenic (cancer-forming) action of any known carcinogen. They also destroy vitamin Bl and can cause nausea and headaches. They can provoke asthma attacks, eczema, hypertension (high blood pressure), and ulcers. I have found they also cause hives or urticaria and in some can result in anaphylactic shock. They appear to reduce levels of calcium in the body, making teeth and bones brittle.

I have found that in several cases they have caused severe coughing in children, which in some instances had been diagnosed as bronchitis by their own doctors. Removing the offending food or drink has resulted in a return to health within days. If you wish to dry your own fruit and vegetables and want to retain the color, dip them in freshly squeezed lemon or pineapple juice.

SODIUM NITRITE AND NITRATE (E 250 AND E 251)

These substances are found in virtually all processed meats, bacon, polony, and Vienna sausages. They interfere with the mechanism for distributing oxygen around the body and they also combine with amines (basic chemicals found in our food) to produce nitrosamines, which are among the most carcinogenic substances ever identified. The question, according to scientists, is not whether they cause cancer but how much cancer they cause.

ACETIC ACID (E 260)

Acetic acid is the main ingredient of vinegar and is thus found in all bottled mayonnaises, dressings, pickles, and sauces. It is used both as a flavorant and a preservative. It is a corrosive and toxic substance that irritates the tissues and can damage the central nervous system, the kidneys, and the liver. Remember that acetic acid is a by-product of fermentation of food in the stomach, frequently the result of poor combining. Using lemon juice on salads is the healthiest option for that tang but if you must use vinegar then grape, apple, or balsamic is best. Read the ingredients; even though vinegar is a natural preservative it often has sulfur dioxide added!

CALCIUM PROPIONATE (E 282)

This is widely used as a preservative in breads, ranging from white loaves to whole wheat and rye. Calcium propionate prevents bread from becoming moldy. It can cause gastrointestinal symptoms similar to a gallbladder attack, and it may also be a cause of migraines. Calcium propionate destroys the enzyme that enables us to assimilate calcium. Imagine a more questionable combination than margarine on bread! So use butter and bake your own bread (or buy from a reputable baker).

The Sweeteners

SORBITOL (E 420)

Sorbitol is mainly used as an artificial sweetener. Formerly presumed safe, recent research shows that there is the possibility of it being carcinogenic, causing, in particular, bladder tumors. It can also produce diarrhea. Sorbitol is not permitted in any baby foods.

ASPARTAME (NO E NUMBER GIVEN AS YET)

Aspartame is also marketed as NutraSweet, Canderel, and various other brand names. Independent scientists claim that aspartame causes mental retardation, brain lesions, and neuroendocrine disorders (disorders associated with the nervous, endocrine, or hormonal systems) thus affecting the thyroid, pituitary, and adrenal glands, the ovaries and testes. In laboratory experiments, lesions (tumors) were produced in the uteruses of rats. According to Professor Wurtman (Massachusetts Institute of Technology) it may also disturb brain function in a variety of ways resulting in epileptic seizures. Further research shows that chronic brain damage may be caused when aspartame is consumed in combination with monosodium glutamate (MSG). Over the years I have dealt with hundreds of women who have had some serious hormonal problems and/or headaches that have cleared up after a few months off sweeteners. Diet soda and sweeteners are not an option in my opinion. Use raw honey or fructose in a powdered form. Other so-called natural sweeteners such as stevia and xylitol are known to cause diarrhea. Xylitol has a bit of a history as some animals in the research inexplicably died. I don't believe either sweetener has been in use long enough to be found safe in humans.

SACCHARIN (NO E NUMBER GIVEN AS YET)

Saccharin has been found to cause cancers in laboratory tests, particularly cancer of the urinary tract. There has been much controversy surrounding this product throughout the past century, but the fact remains that it is carcinogenic and mutagenic.

The most natural sweeteners to use would be freshly extracted fruit juices, dried fruit pastes such as date paste, and raw honey; in small quantities fructose powder can be used as a transitional food because even though it does not upset blood sugar like cane sugar does it is still highly processed and devoid of nutrients.

Miscellaneous Additives

MONOSODIUM GLUTAMATE (NO E NUMBER GIVEN AS YET)

Also known as MSG, this flavor enhancer stimulates the taste buds, which causes them to become inflamed and more sensitive. This deceives us into thinking that foods have more flavor than they really do. MSG is found in packet soups, seasonings, processed savory foods, bouillon cubes, sauces, and almost all fast food. MSG stimulates the taste buds to make them more sensitive which makes the food taste amazing! Just what the fast-food industry wants. In fact, almost every savory processed food contains this chemical and it is often referred to as a *flavor enhancer*. MSG affects the chemistry of the brain, and can cause acute discomfort to the body, including headaches, respiratory problems, and muscle tightness (usually felt in the neck and shoulder area).

CAFFEINE (NO E NUMBER GIVEN AS YET)

Caffeine is found in coffee, cocoa, tea (including green tea), chocolate, and soft drinks. (It is not usually found in herbal teas.) It is a flavoring agent that acts as a stimulant, in turn affecting the central nervous system, the heart, and the kidneys. Consumption can result in nervousness, anxiety, irritability, aggression, sleeplessness, and insomnia. There is strong evidence that caffeine may contribute to the formation of breast lumps. It has also been shown that coffee drinkers are more likely to suffer from heart disease. Continual stimulation of the central nervous system with caffeine can result in tiredness, depression, moodiness, and contributes to ME.

This, by no means, is a comprehensive list of additives. It is merely the tip of the iceberg. It does, however, give you an idea of the additives found most commonly in our foodstuffs.

Irradiation

An additive not generally regarded as such is irradiation or radurization. Irradiation is a preservation treatment that uses very large doses of ionizing radiation, which produces a change in food in order to ensure a longer shelf life. The materials used to irradiate food are cobalt 60 or cesium 137, common nuclear waste products. Irradiation is not new and has been around without our knowledge since 1916 when the first fruit experiments were conducted on strawberries. It is only in the last couple of years that we have become aware of irradiation as more research has appeared in print, and the results of that research are quite alarming. According to Dr. Donald Louria, chairman of the Department of Preventive Medicine and Community Health at the University of Medicine and Dentistry of New Jersey, nuclear waste used in this process takes many years to break down. He claims that research done to date, used as a basis for allowing the irradiation process, was poorly documented. In these experiments, laboratory animals died for no apparent reason. If cats living on a diet of cooked food deteriorate drastically and become sexually deviant and sterile after three generations (according to Dr. F. M. Pottenger in his book *Pottenger's Cats*), how will irradiated foods affect us after a couple of generations? The effects on one generation have not yet been studied satisfactorily. Dr. Louria also states that no irradiation plant is environmentally safe.

Dr. Richard Piccioni, a senior staff scientist with Accord Research, claims that chemical changes take place when food is irradiated so that both known and unknown carcinogens and mutagens are formed in irradiated food. He also says that little research has been done. Dr. George Trisch, a cancer research scientist in Buffalo, New York, says that mutagenic and carcinogenic substances are formed during this process and that formaldehyde (a very toxic substance) is formed in carbohydrates. Dr. Trisch states that in research done on children and animals, more chromosomes appear in the cell (as seen in tumors), and that carcinogenic substances are formed when unsaturated fats are irradiated. Both fruits and vegetables contain carbohydrates and unsaturated fats; therefore, when fruits and vegetables are irradiated, formaldehyde and carcinogenic substances must be formed, resulting in the degeneration of the health of the consumer.

RECAP

The most important thing to remember is that food in its most natural state is best for us. If it has been preserved or colored, has had its flavor enhanced or has been irradiated, we are consuming second-best food. A diet that excludes foods containing additives and includes a high intake of fresh, raw food is the best diet for physical, mental, and emotional well-being. As a safeguard to your family's health, read the ingredients listed on everything you buy. It will cost you nothing and it will preserve your health.

CHAPTER TEN

Exercise, Fresh Air, and Sunshine

IN THIS MODERN DAY and age of high-rise buildings, double-glazing, air-conditioned premises, and artificial lighting, three areas that are often neglected when it comes to health and weight loss are exercise, fresh air, and sunshine. Yet, without ensuring that these three are incorporated in our lives on a daily basis, it would be impossible to achieve and maintain optimum levels of health and weight control. Once again, it is vital to acknowledge the importance of a holistic lifestyle, in other words a lifestyle that includes all those things that pertain to health, not just diet.

Exercise

There is absolutely no way around it—exercise is essential. We are designed to exercise, just as birds are designed to fly. We have more than 400 muscles in our bodies, and as much as we enjoy our modern, labor-saving devices, those muscles were designed to work! So what should we do—throw away our car keys, vacuum cleaners, and washing machines? Well, that would do wonders for the environment, but it is not quite practical in this day and age. What each of us should be doing is finding an exercise program that best suits us and that fits comfortably into our lifestyles.

What sort of exercise, you might ask? An aerobic form of exercise is the most important. Not necessarily a gym aerobics class, but exercising aerobically or "with air." In other words, you should try an exercise that requires you to work your lungs and heart at a steady pace, rather than the stop/start variety. Examples of aerobic exercise are brisk walking, running, cycling, swimming, and gym aerobics.

Of all of these, walking is the most natural form of exercise for man, and you are also less likely to suffer from injuries. An added bonus is that you don't need special shoes or clothing, although flat shoes and loose comfortable clothing are ideal. When I suggest walking, I mean brisk walking that gets your lungs going and your heart pumping. To do this you need to swing your arms and stride out with purpose. Almost anyone can walk. Start by walking around your yard, then around the block. If you're nervous, take a friend or your dog along with you.

What if you don't like walking? Well, find something that you do enjoy. There are plenty of people who have some type of exercise machine hidden away in the depths of the garage. Haul it out! Whatever you do, you must enjoy the exercise, you must feel comfortable, and you must not overdo it. Start slowly and build up your performance and fitness level.

If you are not motivated to exercise on your own, then join an exercise group or a good gym so that you can be monitored. Mark and I enjoy a combination of walking, running, and cycling, whichever takes our mood that day. We particularly enjoy these forms of exercise because we get out into the fresh air. Sundays we like to go for a long, leisurely ride on our bikes and we always took our girls along when they were younger. In between, we garden at least once a week and, believe it or not, we still get stiff! This just goes to show how many of our muscles are under-utilized. We also enjoy a game of tennis or golf when we get an opportunity to play.

Another form of exercise that we enjoy tremendously is rebounding. Jumping on a mini-trampoline or rebounder is an excellent form of aerobic exercise. It is particularly well-suited to confined, indoor areas and is good for when it is raining or if there is not enough time to get out and exercise. You can even do it while you watch the news on television. There is, in fact, no excuse for not exercising in some way or another.

How Much Should You Exercise?

Ideally, you should exercise for no less than twenty minutes a day and preferably between thirty minutes to one hour. If you think you don't have time, you really need just five minutes a day. That's right, all you need is five minutes a day for the first week, and you can build it up slowly to ten minutes a day for the second week. You then continue adding a couple of minutes each week until you've built up to at least twenty minutes a day.

How do you know if you are overdoing it? The best way is to take your pulse. Feel for your heartbeat at the side of your windpipe in your neck, or on the inside of your wrist. Time your heartbeat for fifteen seconds, after fifteen to twenty minutes of exercise. Let's say this figure is twenty-five beats. You multiply this figure by four to find out the beats per minute. For example, 25 x 4 = 100 beats per minute. To find out if you are doing enough work, you subtract your age from 220. Let's say you are forty years old: 220 − 40 = 180. You then multiply that figure by 60 percent to get your minimum heart rate after twenty minutes of exercising: 180 x 60 percent = 108 beats per minute. Your heart at age forty should not beat slower than 108 beats per minute after twenty minutes of aerobic exercise. If it is, then you are not working hard enough. To reach your maximum heart rate, multiply 180 by 85 percent: 180 x 85 percent = 153 beats per minute. At age forty, after twenty minutes of exercise, your heart should not beat faster than 153 beats per minute. If it is, then you are working too hard.

The important points to remember about exercise are that it should be:

- Habitual
- Progressive
- Systematic

HABITUAL

It should become a habit and one of the best ways to form a new habit is to exercise at the same time of the day for at least twenty-one days. This is the time that it takes to either make or break a habit. Exercise at whatever time of the day is most convenient for you. Mark and I enjoy morning exercises, as they really get us in the right frame of mind for the rest of the day.

PROGRESSIVE

Exercise should progress, that is, it should start slowly and easily and steadily increase. It's often very tempting to rush out and exercise madly for an hour, thinking that you will get fit more quickly. You won't. You will probably just end up very tired (and very stiff the next day!) and rather disillusioned.

SYSTEMATIC

Your program should consist of a system of exercises that does three things:

1. Works your lungs, such as running, walking, swimming, and all other forms of aerobic exercise.
2. Stretches your muscles, although it is better to stretch them after you have warmed up. Try touching your toes before and after a workout; you'll get down much further after the workout because your muscles have warmed up.
3. Includes resistance work. No, that's not just weightlifting! Gardening can also be resistance work. A workout in your garden with digging and moving things, such as piles of sand from one place to another, is also good resistance work. Good old push-ups are included here, too. As parents of small children you can get a great workout with your children on the carpet.

Do consult a sports or exercise specialist and read about good resistance and stretching exercises before you begin an exercise regime, as these two types of exercise can lead to injury if incorrectly performed. In fact, it's a good idea to have a check-up with your doctor before you embark on any new exercise program. A good gym will offer you an intensive assessment and is able to refer you to a doctor if any problems arise.

At this point, you might want to know how the Perfect Health dietary program would affect your level of activity. Many sports physiologists have recently found that the most important nutrient in exercise is not protein, as once thought, but rather carbohydrates. Mistakenly, people are encouraged to *carbo-load* on any carbohydrates, including refined carbohydrates. This practice will ultimately cause a loss of nutrients and a drop in blood sugar levels that, in the long term, will impede your performance and damage your health. (For more on this, see chapter five.) Mark and I do a bit of running (our farthest distance being twenty miles). We find that running on an empty stomach is best and we only drink water or a combination of 50 percent pure unsweetened grape juice. The energy we need comes from what we ate one to two days before the run. We find that if we badly combine our food the night before, we feel flat on the day of our run. Similarly, when we eat a refined carbohydrate, especially candy or chocolate, our performance level is adversely affected. I also find that if I eat any dairy products before a run, my stomach and kidneys get quite sore while I'm running. We carbo-load on foods such as bananas, dates, raisins, potatoes, brown rice, and corn on the cob. As for our children, we found that when we exercised with families who ate the "normal way," our children had more endurance. Our grandsons appear to have this same endurance and we have found that their gross motor and fine motor skills are way ahead of their peers. I have also found that every single person I know who follows this program has experienced a vast increase in energy levels and endurance.

Remember that correct nutrition without exercise is not enough, and that vigorous exercise with a bad diet can be dangerous!

Possibly the most important aspect of exercise is that it helps regulate at least eighteen different hormones. These hormones regulate growth hormones, which help correct body weight, slow down the aging process, increase the body's ability to produce energy and break down fat, stabilize blood sugar, and regulate appetite and body temperature, which helps to regulate body weight and appetite. Exercise stimulates endorphins that block pain, make you feel great, and promote a healthy menstrual cycle. It helps to regulate thyroid function, which in turn corrects dry skin, other skin problems, constipation, a fuzzy head, puffy eyes, water retention, lethargy, and regulates your metabolic rate to help correct weight imbalances. Exercise also helps breast-feeding mothers produce sufficient breast milk, and helps prevent and control blood sugar disorders such as diabetes, insulin resistance, and hypoglycemia. Exercise stimulates the production of natural anti-inflammatory chemicals such as cortisol that help deal with inflammatory diseases such as gout, arthritis, and fibromyalgia; exercise helps us efficiently manage stress, improves lung and heart function, and regulates blood pressure.

Regular exercise also helps increase bone density, assisting in the prevention of osteoporosis; it helps regulate reproductive hormones such
as estrogen, progesterone, and testosterone. These are just some of the
main benefits of exercise, and there are plenty more, so if you feel the
need to take something for your health problems, exercise is probably
the most beneficial thing you can take!

Strive for a good balance and whatever you choose to do, get moving
and keep moving.

Fresh Air

More important than any other requirement in life is the air we breathe.
Without air we wouldn't be alive for longer than five to ten minutes. For
this reason, we should try our best to live, dress, and carry ourselves in
a way that does not adversely affect our breathing.

HOMES

We should ensure that we have sufficient ventilation in our homes. In
past consultations, I have often been surprised by the number of people
who sleep with their windows shut. Even if you are worried about se-
curity, try to sleep with a top window open, at least. I have found that
the wider the window is open, the more fresh I feel in the morning. In
winter, even in the coldest climate, Mark and I still sleep with our windows open (even if it is just an inch). We have found in hot states such
as Florida, most families have the air conditioner on and the windows
tightly shut—they are quite shocked that we want the windows open.
There is nothing worse than waking up with a thick head after a night
of inhaling your own carbon dioxide (which is a waste product). If you
have to leave your home unattended during the day, give it a good airing
out every morning by flinging open all doors and windows when you
get up, and then shut them just before you leave. When you get home in
the afternoon, again do the same. If it is cold, dress warmly or put extra
blankets on your bed. If the evening is cool, pull a blanket over your
legs, rather than shutting a window or switching on a heater. To keep
your home fresh and odor-free, good ventilation and plenty of fresh air
are the answers, not cans of "fresh air" spray.

CLOTHING

In order to dress in a manner that does not impede your breathing, you should wear clothes that are loose-fitting. This does not mean that you have to walk around in baggy sacks. Today's fashions allow for loose-fitting, elegant clothes. In fact, you can wear tailored outfits provided that they are not skin-tight. Tight clothing inhibits air circulation and discourages your body from ridding itself of waste products through the skin, resulting in your body becoming toxin-laden and you could end up with skin rashes and clogged lymphatic systems, contributing to lymphatic cancer or lymphoma. Clothing made of natural fibers is the best to wear as these fabrics allow your skin to breathe freely. Natural-fiber clothing is not necessarily more expensive; cotton garments are available from most clothing outlets at reasonable prices. I know it is easier to travel with synthetic fabrics as they are more resistant to creasing, and there is nothing worse than disembarking from a flight appearing as if you've slept under a bush in the park because your one smart linen suit is wrinkled. Make sure at least your underwear is of natural fabric and that the synthetic fabric is not tight-fitting.

POSTURE

Posture is an important factor in receiving sufficient air. To carry yourself in a manner that encourages correct breathing is to walk upright with your shoulders back and your stomach in, just as our mothers have always told us. My mother would make us practice walking across a room with a book on our head, which we thought rather tedious, but I am now grateful that she instilled in us the importance of correct posture. Not only will your breathing be better, but mentally you'll feel ready to take on the world!

To ensure that you get sufficient air at all times, avoid ill-ventilated, stuffy rooms (you don't want to breathe in someone else's waste products), wear comfortable garments made of natural fabrics, and walk tall. I am known to enter talk venues and immediately open the windows. I remember while staying in central Chicago, I could easily see which was my room from the street, even twelve floors up, as it was the only hotel-room window open!

A Little Sunshine

Without sunshine it would be impossible to stay truly healthy; even plants die when they are not exposed to sunlight for some time. Yet the sun has been much maligned and many people avoid it at all costs to the detriment of their health.

One wonders whether this fear of sunshine is not propagated by companies wanting to push their unnatural chemical preparations, such as block-outs, sunscreens, and moisturizers. There have been recent reports that suggest that block-outs and sunscreen creams may cause cancer. This makes sense as the block-out preparations are foreign chemicals that are applied to the skin. I know that in the past when I tried applying these preparations to my own skin, they caused a burning sensation and often resulted in a bit of a rash, even though I tried various respected brands.

The important thing to remember is that the skin is an organ of elimination. If it is continually called upon to eliminate the carcinogenic toxins that we have taken in with our food, then this must be detrimental to the skin. This is especially true of areas exposed to the sun, as the sun speeds up elimination thereby increasing the amount of waste products and toxic substances released through that section of skin. This accelerated process of elimination is the more likely cause of skin cancer.

So, is the sun good or bad for you? The sun is essential for your health and well-being but excessive exposure can be harmful. Your body needs exposure to sunlight so that it can synthesize vitamin D from cholesterol. This, in turn, helps your body to utilize calcium and lowers cholesterol levels. This could be another reason why so many more women than men develop osteoporosis or brittle bones, as they tend to stay out of the sun far more than men, due to the sun's so-called aging effects. Sunlight also affects the number of red cells and hemoglobin in the blood. Too little sunlight results in the serum, or watery portion of the blood, increasing with a proportionate decrease in the red blood cells and fibrin (blood protein) that can cause anemia.

I recall a forty-year-old woman in the medical profession coming to see me. She had been taking iron tablets and had been eating liver for a couple of years, in vast quantities, but to no avail. She remained anemic and her level of health continued to deteriorate. After questioning her about her habits, I found that she worked from 7 A.M. to 8 P.M. every day, often including Saturdays and Sundays. She said that she never had the time to go outside or sit in the sun. Her whole body had a pale, flabby look to it and her skin had an uneven quality. After discontinuing the iron tablets (which were causing constipation) and the liver (which she hated), I corrected her diet and included in her program sunbathing for twenty minutes a day. She had to sit in natural sunlight, exposing as much of her skin as she could for at least twenty minutes a day. Within a month her iron levels were up dramatically, and the overall improvement of her health was significant, as was the quality of her skin and muscle tone.

In addition to its other properties, the sun helps build a better quality of flesh, it enables us to efficiently assimilate food, it stimulates glandular or endocrine activity, it helps with irregularities of ovulation, difficulties in puberty, impotence, acne, psoriasis, nervous disorders including depression, and it also accelerates hair growth and helps to strengthen the eyes as well as improve the quality of sleep.

Obtaining enough light is also of great importance to the pineal gland, a pea-sized gland situated in the brain behind the eyes. This gland is known to regulate both melatonin and serotonin and is considered to be a gland of the endocrine system. It is believed to be important in the role of sexual development in children and other hormonal functions in adults. Melatonin regulation is essential to a good night's sleep. Serotonin is also involved in the sleep process but is known particularly to help us avoid depression. Making sure that you have a minimum of twenty to thirty minutes a day of natural light helps you feel good and sleep well. I have felt the side effects of staying indoors when it is wet and cold. You find you feel tired during the day and sleep poorly at night, either being unable to fall asleep or waking up regularly. This has become a very common problem over the years. We wear sunglasses or shades every second we are outdoors (and some cool dudes even wear them indoors!); most lenses are designed to block ultraviolet rays from your eyes with the mistaken belief that all sunlight, and especially ultraviolet (UV) rays, are bad for our eyes. You need to know that UV rays are essential for the pineal gland to work properly and rather than take medication or drugs to keep you awake during the day, help you sleep at night, and not feel depressed, take half an hour of natural sunlight—it is free, has only positive side effects, and is not addictive!

But as much good as the sun does, it is important not to go out in the periods between about 10 A.M. to 11:30 A.M. and 2:30 P.M. to 4 P.M., depending on the time of year and the cloud coverage. If you don't stay out of the sun at this time of the day, you will certainly damage your skin, as its heat is at its most intense—unless of course it is completely overcast, which can happen even in summer and then even in overcast weather you will benefit more from being outside for half an hour than sitting indoors under artificial light.

Your body, with its innate intelligence, has the built-in ability to tell you that it has had enough sun. This happens when you begin to feel hot, sticky, and uncomfortable. Don't go leaping into a pool to cool down and then get back in the sun, as you will certainly be overdoing it. Twenty minutes to one hour daily is more than enough sunlight to maintain good health without doing damage. If you need to be outside for longer periods for reasons such as watching your child at a sports event, then wear a hat and long, cool sleeves or sit in a shaded area or under an umbrella. Make sure you consume plenty of water to help you cope with fluid loss from the heat, as well.

As far as suntan oils and lotions are concerned, avoid them! They only clog up the pores and prevent the sebaceous or oil glands from correctly functioning, resulting in the skin drying out in the long term. Premature aging and poor texture are sure to occur as a result. If you feel you need a natural moisturizer then use extra-virgin olive oil or extra-virgin coconut oil.

Remember that without regular exercise, a continual supply of fresh air, and a daily dose of sunshine, you cannot begin to achieve or maintain the vibrant health that is your right. Together with a healthy diet these three things have helped Mark and me avoid jet lag on eighteen-hour trans-Atlantic flights!

RECAP

- You need twenty to thirty minutes of exercise daily—start with a few minutes a day and build up as you feel comfortable
- Make sure you are always able to talk while you exercise, but at the same time make sure you sweat or perspire after twenty minutes of exercise
- Ventilate your home daily, even in cold weather
- You need twenty to thirty minutes a day of natural sunlight, and to save time you can get this together with fresh air by exercising outdoors daily. That way you kill three birds with one stone!

CHAPTER ELEVEN

Skin
How to Really Treat It

FOR YEARS I had terribly dry skin. I used some of the top international skin-care brands with no improvement. I slapped on day creams and then night creams and then night creams during the day. My skin became drier and more sensitive. It was only when I changed my diet because of my health problems that I found my skin improved to the point where I have not used skin-care products for more than fifteen years. The one thing people most comment on is how good my skin looks. My husband, Mark, has other *men* lean across the dinner table when we are with friends who ask him what he does to have such great skin. Following the Perfect Health principles not only improves your health and weight—everything starts to function more efficiently, including your skin, hair, and nails.

Much has been written about the skin, there are thousands of skin-care products available, and skin care is a billion-dollar industry. This is another one of the areas where we are bombarded with information based on someone's bottom line and profits. To get some perspective on our skin and how it should be treated, let's start with the basics.

Why Do We Have Skin?

The skin is the largest organ of the body and is mainly an organ of protection. It acts as a shield and protects the body against bacterial and other infections.

Also, the skin is an organ of sensitivity, which enables us to feel various sensations. When you touch something hot your immediate reaction is to withdraw your finger from the heat source. The same thing happens when you go into the sun. After about half an hour you feel hot and uncomfortable. This is because your skin is doing its job as an organ of sensitivity and is sending out warning signals to prevent damage. Listening to your body should apply equally to every part of your body, especially when it comes to your skin and the sun—unless you enjoy looking like a shriveled prune.

The skin is also an organ of elimination, which simply means that it provides the body with a mechanism to cleanse itself. A simple skin rash is often nothing more than an indication that the body is eliminating something foreign or toxic and this process results in inflammation of the skin. I find, for example, that I get hives or urticaria (a type of skin rash) from a particular additive that is used in some chocolates and from sulfur dioxide, a preservative widely used in foods and drinks. My skin becomes extremely inflamed and itchy and this may be my body trying to excrete the offending substance. In the beginning, I would traipse off to the doctor for some type of anti-inflammatory medication, but it never made much difference. With or without medication it would take at least two weeks to clear up. With a change in my diet and plenty of foods high in essential fatty acids (Omega 3 and Omega 6—see chapter eight) it seldom takes longer than two to three days to completely clear and does not flare up to the extent it used to.

More often than not, a rash or similar skin condition is caused by incorrect eating. By rectifying this, most skin conditions clear. The severe dermatitis on my hands that I suffered from totally cleared up within four days of combining my food correctly, and would then reappear when I went back to eating protein and starches at the same meal. This condition could have many causes such as the alcohol, acetic acid, or ammonia from incompletely digested protein, or even histamines that are formed when food ferments in the stomach because of incorrect combinations. These toxic substances are then excreted through the skin. This generally affects those people with sensitive skin. The body uses one of the other excretory organs (lungs, bowels, kidneys, and bladder) in those people not susceptible to skin problems.

As I mentioned, your skin is an excretory organ. It is therefore important that you drink plenty of water every day as this will help to flush impurities from your body that would otherwise be excreted by the skin. Natural spring water is the best option. (See chapter twelve.)

Skin is also an organ of nutrition because it synthesizes vitamin D from the sun. Vitamin D is an important nutrient that plays a role in maintaining calcium levels and phosphorus metabolism in the body. Vitamin D is also thought to play a role in iron assimilation; this is one of the reasons low iron levels or anemia that results in pale skin can be corrected with half an hour of natural light exposure. Vitamin D has recently been seen as an important factor in immune function as it appears to protect against cancer, including skin and prostate cancer and autoimmune diseases such as multiple sclerosis, diabetes, and arthritis. Yet more reason to spend those twenty to thirty minutes a day outdoors.

How Should You Really Treat Your Skin?

The most important way to treat your skin is to eat correctly. Never before has the old adage "you are what you eat" been truer than when it is applied to the skin. I have dealt with many people whose skin has benefited tremendously by correcting their eating habits. My "dry, sensitive" skin is now far more "balanced" and the most dramatic change came about when I started eating a predominantly raw fruit and vegetable diet, making sure to include essential fatty acids, exclude gluten from my diet, and also include dark green leafy vegetables (for me this is my extracted organic dried barley grass juice).

I investigated body brushing as an alternative to soap and for many years now I have used no soap on any part of my body. My skin is softer and cleaner than it has been in years! Although I do still use a natural glycerine bar of soap to wash my hands after going to the bathroom or if I inadvertently get grease from my bicycle chain on my hands or legs when I have been for a ride.

As soap is alkaline, it counteracts the natural acidity of the skin, which has a pH level of about 5.5. This results in an alkaline environment, ideal for the proliferation of bacteria. You will find that sores and scratches heal much quicker when you stop stripping off your acid mantle and follow a diet that encourages a healthy immune system. Washing with soap also removes natural oils from the surface of the skin, leaving it dry and taut, dead skin cells remain behind on the skin's surface, resulting in that flaky, dry look. So you have your natural oils stripped off to encourage an alkaline environment ideal for bacterial growth with plenty of food for the bacteria in the form of dead skin cells! Body brushing with a loofah or natural bristle brush—not nylon, which will damage your skin—on the other hand, keeps both the pH balance and the natural oils intact, yet removes the dead skin cells from the surface, resulting in softer, smoother, and healthier skin.

Since I stopped using soap, I have not needed any moisturizer, sun block, sunscreen, or hand and body lotion, yet my skin is now in peak condition. No more burning cheeks, dry legs and hands, or cracked heels for me! Ask yourself, does it make sense to remove your natural oils and then to replace them with an artificial chemical or even so-called natural, herbal mixture?

It is only because of years and years of eating the foods that our systems were not designed to consume that our skin starts to act up and give us trouble. Add to that excessive exposure to very strong sunlight and artificial skin preparations and you have the answer to premature aging of the skin.

If you have never brushed your body, now is the time to start! Bristle brushing can be done either on dry skin before you bathe, as the Europeans suggest (brushing with firm strokes toward the heart), or in the bath or shower as others prefer. I suggest you only brush your body once a day, preferably in the morning as this is when there are the most dead skin cells on the surface of your skin. During the night while you sleep, your skin replaces old cells at two-and-a-half times the rate it normally does during the day. (Remember the body cycles and how your body repairs more while you sleep.)

Use firm movements and do not keep brushing the same spot for too long. You will only damage your skin, as I have, and you will end up with red, angry skin and can even bleed. You will also find that with body brushing, lymphatic drainage is encouraged and this will encourage cellulite to disappear in time. The same diet that results in good health will forever get rid of your cellulite. Another benefit of following Perfect Health!

As for my face, I brush with a loofah or a soft bristle brush (a shaving brush can be used although I prefer something a bit firmer). I do this in the mornings only. Remember to be gentle with the skin on your face. At night I use a clean cotton face-cloth with warm water. If I wear makeup, I remove it with water. I choose water-soluble organic makeup products that are not tested on animals.

Don't expect overnight miracles; your skin will not suddenly become soft and dewy in a day or even a month. It took time for you to get your skin out of balance, and it will take time—from a few months to one or two years—to get it working like it should. It did take about a year to wean myself off all creams and for my own skin to achieve an optimum balance by producing just enough oil to prevent either oiliness or dryness. I achieved this by applying creams less and less frequently—from once a day to once every two days, until I used creams only on days that my skin was a bit too dry. Eventually I found that I could go without any skin-care products at all and now only use a little extra-virgin olive or coconut oil when necessary. My skin can feel especially dry when I swim in summer, fly, or if I am exposed to indoor heating for an extended period of time.

If you are using a skin-care line, change to an organic 100 percent natural one that contains no animal products or artificial colorants and preservatives. Also support one that does not test on animals and use a pH-balanced cleanser on the rest of your body. (Visit www.mary-anns.com for what I recommend.)

I was recently shocked to discover that the average lipstick-wearing woman consumes two tubes of lipstick each year, just from licking her lips and being kissed. (Where do you think all that lipstick disappears to?) The average lipstick has some very damaging chemicals in it, including post-slaughter products from animals.

If you wear make up, always remove it before going to bed at night. It is important that you clean your skin well at night as this is the time your body steps up repair work and leaving makeup on the skin will hinder this process.

Olive oil is a great makeup remover. Use a cotton ball to remove all traces of mascara, especially waterproof mascara. Blot off excess oil with a tissue or tone with a little diluted apple cider vinegar if you don't like the oily residue on your skin. There are now special makeup removal face cloths—one of them called the "Magic Mitt." I use this daily and it is truly magic as it removes even heavy makeup with a few swipes after being dipped in warm water!

Eating for Healthy Skin

If your diet is healthy and your body is working in perfect harmony, then this will be reflected through your skin. The moment that something in your body is out of balance, one of the first signs will be the lack of luster evident in your eyes and in your skin. Considering that skin function is controlled by the endocrine (hormonal) system it would make sense to eat foods that help this hormonal system work more efficiently. Most skin problems result when this delicate system is out of balance.

Any and all foods that affect the endocrine system will either positively or negatively affect the skin. As in so many other areas of hormonal function, refined sugar is particularly disruptive to the skin and so is gluten (the protein found in wheat, oats, rye, and barley), which can cause either dry or oily skin, or even acne. (By the way, gluten is found only in the grains of these plants and not the leaves, so rest assured that barley grass or wheat grass juice is gluten-free!)

Your coloring is determined by the amount of melanin that is produced by your skin. Melanin absorbs UV rays and acts as a natural sunscreen. Your diet can help to sustain and even increase your melanin production, thereby ensuring greater protection against the sun's harmful rays. Eating regular amounts of orange and yellow fruits and vegetables, such as mangoes and carrots, will provide the nutrients (especially beta-carotene) that help perform this function and protect you from skin cancer. You will find your skin developing a distinct yellow undertone when you eat more fruit and vegetables; this is totally harmless and proves that you are developing natural protection from skin cancer. If you would like to rid your skin of that yellow undertone, simply spend thirty minutes a day exposing your skin to natural sunlight and you will develop a healthy, even glow!

Although everybody has different skin, there are three main classifications of skin types and most people have either one or a combination of these: normal; dry/sensitive; oily. Many people, particularly teenagers, have combination skin. The forehead, nose, and chin form an oily "T" area, while the rest of the face is dry.

If you realize that the skin is controlled by the hormonal system and that everything you eat has either a positive or a negative effect on this hormonal system, then it is easier to understand how diet affects the skin.

The issue is not how to eat according to your skin type but to know that depending on your genetic makeup, your skin could become dry and sensitive because of your diet, but your spouse or children may have oily skin from exactly the same foods. That is probably why people cannot make the connection, as on the same diet different people's skin responds in different ways.

Everything you eat and drink will have an effect on this system. We know that the hormonal system must have essential fatty acids, plenty of vitamins and minerals (from fresh fruits and vegetables, not tablets) to function optimally, but what we don't realize is that heated fats and fried foods such as fast food, margarine, and coffee and tea creamers prevent your body from utilizing those essential fatty acids and in so doing upset the hormonal system. Your skin may respond to this by "breaking out" in pustules, becoming dry and sensitive, or simply by aging faster.

Gluten does contribute to skin problems and I have seen that when people remove gluten from their diets for a period of at least six weeks, their skin responds beautifully. I know that within twenty-four hours of eating wheat or rye my skin is itchy and dry. My daughters Melissa and Meredith will respond with pimples on their chins and foreheads, Marie-Claire will have pimples on the back of her upper arms and her butt, and Mark will get pimples on his upper thighs and nose. As you can see, even in the same family each person can have a different response. Spots or pimples on the back of your upper arms and cracked heels are common in gluten intolerant people and so it is best to remove these foods. Gluten has now been found to cause severe problems with the hormonal system, including autoimmune diseases and infertility, so it makes sense that it can cause problems with other systems controlled by the hormonal system, such as skin.

Gluten, refined sugar, and the protein in dairy products (milk, yogurt, and cheese) are also known to be major factors in eczema as is a lack of essential fats. So remove all dairy products and include natural fats for at least six weeks to see a change.

Replace gluten-containing starches with potatoes, millet, quinoa, sweet potatoes, yams, corn, and brown (unrefined) rice.

Skin problems can also be caused by not drinking enough water and by consuming caffeine through tea, coffee, chocolates, or sodas. Yes, chocolate can cause skin problems contrary to what your dermatologist may tell you. Chocolate contains three ingredients that upset the hormonal system: caffeine, refined sugar, and cow's milk.

Avoid coffee, tea (including green tea as it contains caffeine and it is

better to obtain the bioflavenoids and antioxidants claimed to be of benefit in green tea from caffeine-free fresh fruit and vegetables), chocolate,
and any drinks or foods that contain caffeine, sweeteners, and refined
sugar as they tend to upset the hormonal system and can affect your
skin. Be aware of certain herbal teas that claim to stimulate the kidneys,
as these also cause you to lose excess fluid. Replace them with fruit and
caffeine-free herbal teas, carob bars and drinks, and freshly extracted
fruit juices or 100 percent pure fruit juices that you can dilute.

It is vital that you eat plenty of red (such as beets, tomatoes, or strawberries), green (barley grass or wheat grass juice, spinach, herbs such as
rocket and basil), and orange fruit and vegetables daily as these provide
essential antioxidants that prevent your skin from becoming over-ex-
posed to pollutants in the air. Barley grass is the most nutritious of these
foods and does not contain oxalic acid like spinach does. Oxalic acid
prevents you from efficiently using the iron and calcium in spinach.

Refined sugar and alcohol play havoc with the endocrine (hormonal)
system and can therefore cause a variety of skin problems. The only reason dermatologists would tell you that sugar or diet does not affect your
skin is because they study diseases of the skin and how to treat them
with medication, and have not studied diet and the role it plays. They
generally and incorrectly conclude that because diet was not included
in their curriculum, it is not a factor in skin problems. Diet is a major
factor when it comes to skin and the sooner you make the changes, the
sooner you, too, will have glowing skin. In the process, you will probably save a considerable amount of money, too! Remember that artificial
sweeteners added to foods or in diet sodas also upset the hormonal system, so replace refined sugar with raw honey and fructose or dried and
fresh fruit for natural sweetness in your diet.

Smoking cigarettes probably does more damage to the skin than any
other bad habit. Smoking starves the skin of many nutrients such as
oxygen and B-complex vitamins (to name a few), resulting in a gray,
dull, slack appearance. Without fail, I can pinpoint the smokers just by
the tone and color of their skin. Besides upsetting the hormonal system, cigarettes, caffeine, and alcohol contribute to tiny blood capillar-
ies under the skin bursting, which you see on the cheeks and noses of
some people. Remember that by combining your food badly, alcohol is
formed in the digestive tract. It then gets into the bloodstream and is
transported throughout the body, including the skin. Just eating concentrated protein and starches at separate meals can improve your skin

condition considerably, as can not smoking or consuming alcohol and caffeine-containing drinks and foods.

Exercise is of great benefit to the skin as it gets the heart pumping faster. This, in turn, gets more nutrients speedily to the skin and achieves that healthy glow. Exercise also has a profound effect on the hormonal system that benefits the skin. (See chapter ten.) Fresh air and sunshine also have a vital role to play. I find that being in an air-conditioned or heated room dries the skin out terribly.

So you don't have to spend a fortune on your skin after all. With the correct diet and sensible habits, including regular exercise, fresh air, and sunshine, you can have healthy, glowing skin for life.

There are many other factors that influence skin type, and apart from the obvious ones such as heredity, climate, and age, several others including medications (such as contraceptive pills), air-conditioning, artificial heating, and stress also play a part.

You will find, though, that with a natural diet, exercise, and fresh air, even with these other factors your skin can considerably improve.

I think it is vital that you take the most natural route possible when it comes to skin care, especially when it comes to correcting certain problems such as acne, dermatitis, or eczema. The more you turn to prescription medications, the more you expose your body to harmful side effects. If you insist on taking medication, make sure you are 100 percent aware of all the possible side effects by reading the insert or going onto the drug company's Web site. But I would strongly urge you to change your diet as suggested above, rather than go on medication, so that you treat the cause and not just the symptom.

RECAP

- Following Perfect Health will help your hormonal system function efficiently and this is the system that controls your skin
- Start with the five steps
- Clean your skin with a natural bristle brush or cotton cloth and avoid using soap
- Remove caffeine, alcohol, sugar, artificial sweeteners, gluten, dairy products, heated fats, and cigarettes from your diet
- Include natural plant fats in your diet on a daily basis
- Exercise daily

- Make sure you obtain fresh air and natural light on a daily basis; exercising outdoors would help you achieve this
- In time you, too, will have people leaning across the dinner table asking how you have such beautiful skin!

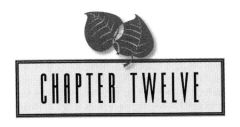

CHAPTER TWELVE

Water
How Much, How Often, What Type?

I LIKE TO THINK of water as the forgotten nutrient as we are seldom alerted to its importance. We seem to know a great deal about the vitamins and minerals that sustain our health, yet without water we would simply not be able to utilize any of these nutrients effectively. As our bodies are made up of approximately 60 percent water, it is perhaps the single most important nutrient. It is often the most neglected one, too.

Why Do We Need Water?

Dehydration can have a serious impact on your physical health and mental well-being. The central nervous system is the first to show functional changes when the body is not sufficiently hydrated. One of the first signs is usually tiredness (constant yawning), followed by a headache and an inability to concentrate. Thirst and dryness of the mouth will alert you to the fact that you need to increase your fluid intake, but if you ignore these messages, other symptoms will soon manifest. These include uncooperative or sullen behavior, weakness, and lassitude, and at a later stage, mental confusion. In severe cases the cheeks become pale and the lips dry and blue; the skin loses its elasticity; the eyeballs have a sunken appearance and dark circles appear under them; and loss of weight is not uncommon. Dehydration during prolonged exercise (after more than one hour) encourages cardiovascular drift—a condition where the heart beats faster but less blood is pumped out. This obviously puts tremendous strain on the heart and should be avoided at all costs.

It is interesting that the first thing we reach for when we are tired is usually caffeine in some form or another—tea, coffee, sodas, or chocolate—but this just contributes to further dehydration because more fluid is needed to expel the toxins from the cells. For every glass of dehydrating fluid (and that includes that refreshing glass of beer on a hot summer's day!) you need to drink one or two glasses of pure, clean water to ensure that your body remains hydrated at the cellular level. A pint (half a liter) of clean, filtered, or natural spring water on your desk will help you consume the minimum intake of water that you daily require.

But learn to listen to your body—simply forcing water down your throat for the sake of it will put unnecessary strain on your kidneys. New research by Professor Tim Noakes of the Sports Science Institute in Cape Town, South Africa, indicates that over-hydration (or hyponatraemia) is no joke. It causes the body and brain to swell and this can lead to convulsions, heart failure, and the cessation of breathing, as well as fluid retention. So drink only when you are thirsty and not because someone has told you that you need to down eight or ten glasses of water a day.

How Much Water Do We Need?

As water is so vital to our physical health and mental well-being it makes sense that our diet should contain a high percentage of water. We need at least five to six glasses of water every day to ensure that we meet the body's basic fluid requirements. The more raw fruits and vegetables you consume the less water you will need to drink, but the more protein and processed foods you consume the more water you will need. People on a 70–80 percent raw food diet (which is ideal for vibrant health) find that they tend to drink less water as their diet provides most of the fluid they need. Very few people manage this, however, so you should aim at drinking between five to six glasses of water daily.

There will be times when you need more water than others. We need to increase our water intake when we are sick (when we are running a temperature, have excessive mucus discharge, or if we are suffering from diarrhea, for example). We also need more water when we are exercising or if we lose a lot of fluid through perspiration. If your diet is not as healthy as it should be, particularly if you eat animal protein more than once a day, your body will require more water to function properly.

Generally the best advice I can offer is that you should drink a glass of water if you are thirsty, and only then have a hot or cold beverage if you still feel like it. I am constantly amazed at parents who tell me that their children will not drink water. The only reason for this, I believe, is that these children were not given water right from the word *go*. If you are one of those people who hate water try adding 100 percent pure juices such as Ceres to flavor it. You can also use the juices to make ice cubes and add them to your water—children in particular will more readily drink water with juice-colored ice cubes. Just make sure the juices are genuinely pure and contain no additives (such as sugar or preservatives).

The body is designed to quench its thirst with water and this is what should always be first offered. I would go so far as to say that when you feel hungry, drink a glass of water before you reach for something to eat. Very often we confuse the signals for hunger and thirst and you might find that your hunger pangs are nothing more than plain thirst, after all. Decide if you still really need to eat only after you have drunk a glass of water. This will also help you learn to interpret correctly the body's signals.

Water is an essential component of both protoplasm and blood. Cells must be bathed in fluid at all times to do their work, so correct hydration is vitally important at the cellular level. Cancer is thought by some to be the result of continual dehydration at this basic cellular level.

The body relies on water to flush away waste products such as urine. Without water to moisten the surface of the lungs, there can be no intake of oxygen or expulsion of carbon dioxide. For food to be digested, absorbed, and carried to all parts of the body, water is needed every step of the way. In fact, even if you are eating sufficiently, dehydration (or a lack of sufficient water) can lead to malnutrition.

Water is essential for temperature maintenance, for many chemical reactions in the body, and for lubrication and protection of joint surfaces. It also helps to maintain the necessary pressure in certain parts of the body, such as the eyeballs. And, of course, it is responsible for

maintaining comfortable levels of lubrication in the eyes and for producing tears.

Muscles consist of 75 percent water and therefore need this vital fluid
to relax and contract efficiently and to maintain strength and tone. Good
muscle tone protects your body and muscle activity helps to strengthen
your bones. Water is also necessary for keeping the skin supple and
elastic—dehydration can contribute to the aging process.

Water is vital for effective brain function. In fact, many courses on
maximizing your brain capacity encourage you to drink a glass of water
at least every hour, as dehydration can lead to mental confusion and
emotional stress and is detrimental to retaining information (memory).
A high fruit- and vegetable-based diet, as advocated in this book, will
result in more efficient brain function partially due to the high water
content of fresh fruit and vegetables.

The endocrine system, which influences every aspect of our health
and well-being, is totally reliant on water for almost every chemical
reaction. With adequate water, all the systems in your body work at
optimum levels to the benefit of your health.

The hypothalamus, situated in the brain, regulates the conservation,
replenishment, and elimination of water. It links the nervous system
to the endocrine system (hormones) by synthesizing and secreting
neurohormones, as needed by the body, that control the secretion of
hormones from the anterior pituitary gland—among them, gonadotro-
pin-releasing hormones (GnRH). The neurons that secrete GnRH are
linked to the limbic system, which is primarily involved in the control
of emotions and sexual activity. The hypothalamus also controls body
temperature, hunger, thirst, and circadian rhythms.

These processes can be affected by the quantity and type of water we
drink since inorganic mineral deposits can impair the functioning of the
hypothalamus and can easily damage the thyroid, adrenal, and pituitary
glands. Inorganic minerals are brought into the body by water that has a
high mineral content. Drinking water that has a pH of between 6.8 and 7.2
will avoid this problem; outside of this range the body struggles to deal with
the mineral imbalance as it is designed to use water at a pH of 7.

About three-quarters of the body fluid is stored within the cells, and
without water, cells would literally shrivel up and die. Blood plasma,
which transports mineral salts, carbohydrates, proteins, gases, enzymes,
fats, and hormones, is approximately 92 percent water. All the nutrients
that we take into our bodies are ultimately broken down to become wa-

ter-soluble. In other words, they are able to dissolve in water. The whole aim of the digestive process is to break food down so that it dissolves easily in water. In this way the nutrients can be transported throughout the system by the blood. Drinking during a meal does not facilitate this process. It tends to dilute the digestive enzymes in the stomach so that the food is then not easily broken down. This can also result in fermentation, even though the meal might be properly combined. It is best to drink half an hour before the meal, or one to two hours after the meal.

Which Water Is Best?

Tap water is contaminated with many harmful substances (for instance, it picks up heavy metals such as lead in older piping systems). It is chlorinated to kill bacteria and hopefully neutralize fecal matter, but the chlorine combines with naturally occurring organic substances, forming highly carcinogenic trihalomethanes or chlorinated hydrocarbons. Chlorine has been found to contribute to arteriosclerosis (hardening of the arteries), asthma attacks, nausea, and disorientation. In addition, chlorine is a powerful irritant that also destroys vitamin E and because of its sterilizing properties destroys vitamin B12. Vitamin E is a natural antioxidant that helps prevent cancer and vitamin B12 is essential for healthy nerves and brain.

We are designed to deal comfortably with water that has a neutral pH level, as it neither leaches minerals from the body (as a more acidic pH will do) nor leaves behind inorganic mineral deposits (as is the case with water that is too alkaline). Mineral loss can contribute to osteoporosis and heart disease, and inorganic mineral deposits are associated with kidney stones and have been linked to stiffening joints and arthritis. Ideally water should have a pH not greater than 7.2 and not less than 6.8. You will find that water at this pH level actually tastes sweet and quenches your thirst adequately.

Fluoride has been found to stimulate bone formation, but the bones become poorly mineralized and brittle. Fluoride is also toxic to the rest of the body. Dr. Leo Spiro, who was awarded a degree in recognition for his research on fluoridation by London University, says that fluoride damages brain and nerve cells, is harmful to reproductive organs, affects the thyroid gland, damages the liver, and creates a high incidence of bone fracture. He adds that, "We cannot prophecy what would happen to the organs of the body if it were subjected to constant doses of fluoride for a lifetime." Fluoride is one of those industrial waste products that someone decided would be of benefit, without having done any long-term tests on the effects it would have on the human body. It really is about profit, not health!

There is not much you can do at the point of purification, but at least you can do something about the quality of the water in your own home. You can easily filter your water by using any of the variety of filter systems currently available. For the most part, they are practical and easy to use, and they remove chlorine, heavy metals such as mercury, lead, cadmium, arsenic, and organic contaminants from the water. As there are many domestic water-purification systems on the market, I suggest that you look for an established brand, backed by solid research, which will be able to supply you with replacement filters or cartridges for years to come. Ultimately, all drinking water should be filtered, and so should any water that you use for cooking.

Reverse osmosis is a wasteful way of purifying water and, just as with distilling water, it strips the water of all minerals, resulting in an acidic pH. If the water is too alkaline these naturally occurring organic minerals can contribute to kidney stones and stiffening of the joints as the body is unable to deal with the excess, and if the water is too acidic your body will need extra alkaline minerals such as calcium, magnesium, and potassium to return the water to its neutral pH. The body will obtain these alkaline minerals from your bones and this will contribute to osteoporosis.

Another indicator that the water is too high in these inorganic minerals is a high TDS (Total Dissolved Solids) and it is best to drink water with a TDS less than 100.

Although bottled water is often rich in minerals, unfortunately these minerals are not present in a form that our bodies are able to easily use. Unlike the minerals in fresh fruits and vegetables, those in mineral water are easily deposited in our joints, muscles, and tissues, where they can cause stiffness, gall or kidney stones, premature aging of the skin, and even cataracts. Therefore, it is therefore important to make sure bottled water has a pH that is as close to neutral (7) as possible. Do not be alarmed. This does not mean that you should never touch bottled water—it is probably the best type of drink you could have in a social situation. If you have a choice, go for the non-carbonated variety, as the bubbles in sparkling mineral water are formed by carbon dioxide, a waste product that the body tries to eliminate. It doesn't make sense to force carbon dioxide into the body when it has gone to so much trouble to get rid of it in the first place. But, at the end of the day, carbonated water is better than most other drinks on the market and is still a better choice than alcohol or other sweetened drinks.

Tips for Healthy Hydration

Water is vital for your health. If you want to take full control of your physical and mental well-being it is important to include this precious fluid in your daily routine.

- When you are thirsty, let your first choice be a glass of filtered water
- At work keep a large bottle of fresh, clean water on your desk
- At home keep a water filter jug (see www.mary-anns.com for ones I personally recommend) or a bottle of natural spring water in your refrigerator
- Carry a water bottle with you when you leave the house (some filters also come in a handy sports bottle that you can fill at any tap to be assured that you are getting pure, filtered water at a fraction of the cost of bottled water)
- Avoid beverages containing caffeine (coffee and sodas)
- Drink herbal infusions instead of Ceylon (black) or green tea
- Avoid sodas and diet drinks (they contain many harmful additives and sweeteners)
- Drink natural fruit juices instead (diluted with sparkling mineral water if you miss the fizz)
- For every caffeinated beverage you drink, have a glass of pure water
- Sip a glass of water slowly before eating meals and snacks
- Reduce the amount of alcohol you consume—aim at eliminating it altogether, but at least drink a glass of filtered or bottled water with, before, or after each alcoholic beverage
- Order bottled water in restaurants
- Add a slice of lemon or lime to your water or even a touch of pure fruit juice (such as grape juice) if it helps you to enjoy water more
- Make sure you follow the Perfect Health five steps so that you are eating a high water content diet. This will go a long way to alleviating many symptoms related to dehydration

RECAP

- Before you drown in all these details, remember that you should listen to your body when it comes to drinking water
- When thirsty, drink clean, filtered, or spring water
- A diet high in fresh raw fruit and vegetables is able to supply a great deal of the water your body needs
- Remember that fruit, our ideal food, contains as much as 80–90 percent pure water
- If you need to drink socially, go for natural, unsweetened, preservative-free fruit juices or mineral waters
- Try to leave out the fizz if you can. But even with the bubbles, these choices are still better than any of the artificially sweetened and processed sodas on the market. (Try not to drink more than one glass of commercial fruit juice in a day. They are heated to kill bacteria and in the process become quite acidic to the body. A number of the nutrients are also destroyed by this process)
- Pure water always comes out on top. A glass of water with a slice of lemon not only tastes good, but looks fashionable, too. Cheers!

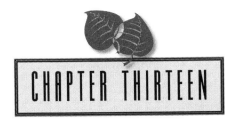

CHAPTER THIRTEEN

Fasting and Detoxification
Ways to Supreme Health

NO, FASTING IS NOT confined to religious fanatics, it just happens to be one of the fastest ways to supreme health, well-being, and optimum weight levels—if done in a well-planned, informed way. Fasting is not dangerous and has been done for centuries by people of all walks of life.

True fasting means eating nothing at all, drinking only pure water, and resting both physically and mentally. Rest is what a fast is all about. A true fast allows the body and mind to rest completely and redirect energy toward healing and correcting any problems that may exist. Complete rest is vitally important when fasting as it restores the body physically, emotionally, mentally, and spiritually. The ideal setting should be a quiet place away from family, work, television, radio, and the general hustle and bustle of everyday life. The last thing you need during a fast is stress of any description. The mind and body must be in a state of repose or rest.

The benefits of fasting are tremendous. Your general health improves, your skin and eyes glow, and you feel as if you've had a total "overhaul" or body-lift. A properly supervised fast, followed by a correct eating program, is one of the best and quickest ways to glowing health. If you are looking for an extreme make-over then this is the quickest, cheapest, and safest! Honestly, the effect of fasting on the skin and body is quite miraculous.

People often refer to abstaining from solid foods but drinking juice as a *juice fast*. This is, in fact, not a fast at all, but a diet—a juice diet to be exact.

A *Daniel fast* is not a fast, either; chapter one of the Old Testament *Book of Daniel* tells of him in captivity and how he refused to eat the king's rich foods; rather he and three other young men chose to eat only vegetables (or plant food) and water. To make sure they were not starving, the chief in charge of the young men checked after ten days to see how they had done and they "were looking better and had taken on more flesh than all the youths who ate of the king's dainties" (Dan 1:15). This prompted the chief to feed the same diet to all the other youths. So this is clearly no fast as these young men became stronger on this diet; in fact, the diet is very similar to Perfect Health! If you feel the need to detoxify your body then a diet of just plant food for a few weeks every six months is a very good idea—you may feel so good by eating just plant food that you do not want to go back to your old, flesh-eating ways!

There is only one kind of fast and that is a total abstinence from nourishment of any kind. Even taking in honey or grapefruit juice does not make it a true fast.

During a fast, the body redirects the energy it would otherwise use for digesting meals and other daily activities to any problem area in the body. In other words, the body is given an opportunity to focus on cleansing and healing. Weight loss is also achieved more quickly on a fast as the body burns any excess fat deposits for fueling its normal functions. (The average weight loss is from 1–2 pounds per day.)

A word of caution is needed here. Fasting for more than two to three days should not be embarked on without the guidance of a health counselor or someone who has both studied and undergone a fast him or herself. Do not rush into a fast. It is essential that you are adequately prepared for the fast and properly supervised while fasting. If you are pregnant, lactating, or on any medication you should be extremely cautious and if you feel the need to fast under these circumstances, then it is best to be monitored by a trained counselor. If you plan to fast even with the aid of a counselor, read as much as you can on the subject before you begin. Ideally, you should eat only raw foods for as many days before and after as days you are on the fast. In other words, if you are planning a two-day fast, stick to raw foods for two days before you begin and continue with raw foods for two days after. You don't start fasting because you have over-indulged and want to punish yourself. A fast must be planned carefully; fasting employed correctly can result in the body performing miracles. I have seen this not only in myself, but in many other people, as well.

Take the case of Ingrid, age twenty-one. Ingrid was diagnosed as having a cyst close to her anus and was told that her only option was surgery. Ingrid chose instead to fast; she was worried that a slip of the knife might cause problems with passing waste products or having a child in the future. She started by only eating fruit for a week before the fast; this was to ensure that there was no fermenting, old food in her digestive tract as she went into the fast and to ensure that she had gone through some of the detoxification prior to the fast, which would speed up the healing process during the fast. She then embarked on a true fast, i.e., no food or juices—just clean, fresh water. By the fifth day of the fast, Ingrid reported that her urine and body odor smelled very strongly of Roaccutane. This is a so-called "miracle drug" that was prescribed for her skin the previous year at an exorbitant cost for a six-month treatment. Ingrid was warned at the time that she should not become pregnant for at least a year, as the drug could damage the fetus. (Some suggest that this period should be five years.) All that the drug seemed to achieve was to dehydrate her nasal passages, eyes, and skin terribly. Ingrid said that her urine continued to have this odor for a couple more days and that by the eighth day of the fast, the cyst had broken down completely. She then broke her fast by drinking freshly extracted fruit juice, and continued to eat fruit and raw vegetables, until she gradually introduced cooked vegetables and carbohydrates. Now, sixteen years later, the cyst has not reappeared. Ingrid has gone on to marry, have a child, and raise him on Perfect Health; she has studied the Natural Health Course as well as the Consulting Course and helps people correct their lifestyles.

Sandy, on the other hand, age thirty-eight, had numerous complaints. She suffered from a candida (a type of yeast infection) overgrowth that resulted in severe digestive problems. Her stomach bloated virtually every time she ate something. (candida usually results from use of antibiotics, contraceptive pills, and a diet that is high in processed and refined foods.) Even after changing her diet to the Perfect Health program, Sandy still battled with the candida, although there was an improvement in her general health. Encouraged by her doctor, Sandy embarked on a supervised fasting program. She was able to take time off work and managed to fast, very comfortably I might add, for sixteen days (and she would have fasted longer, but she needed to return to work). Sandy had a medical check-up, including blood tests, before and after the fast. Before the fast, her doctor said that her liver was not functioning properly, that she could not assimilate or absorb potassium effectively, and that she had the previously mentioned candida problem. After the fast her potassium levels were corrected, her liver was functioning 100 percent, and the candida problem had cleared up.

Fasting, as can be seen from these case studies, is to be taken seriously and should not be undertaken on a whim. Although fasting for one day a week or once a month is easily achievable and can give the digestive tract a good rest, anything longer should be supervised by an experienced consultant. The duration of your fast depends on your general state of health, your fat reserves, and on whoever is supervising you. There have been cases where severely obese people have fasted for up to three months, and then there are other frequent cases where individuals should not fast for more than a day or two. One of the best books to read that will help you is *Fasting and Eating for Health: A Medical Doctor's Program for Conquering Disease* by Joel Fuhrman, M.D.

Fasting for a day or two before changing your diet is also a good way to kick-start you into a correct eating program. This way you make a clean start and after a fast, all that fresh, raw food tastes so good! It is also one of the quickest ways I have seen people quit smoking. I have yet to discover anyone who can fast and still smoke at the same time. Your body is also able to rid itself of the toxins from smoking far more quickly during a fast, and once the fast is broken there is no craving for the taste of tobacco.

I am deliberately not going into too much detail on fasting in this chapter, as I merely wish to point you in the right direction and ensure that you find a person who has experience with fasting to help you. (Fasting is a subject that requires a book of its own!) In the last few years, I have been able to train many people in the principles of fasting, who are now Perfect Health consultants and are listed on www.mary-anns.com.

Detoxification

One of the main reasons that you should find someone to monitor your fast is that the symptoms of detoxification that usually accompany a fast can be unpleasant. These symptoms can include headaches, migraines, dizziness, nausea, dry mouth, muscle cramps, sores in the mouth, and a strong, unpleasant body odor. These symptoms are unpleasant and can be very frightening if you do not know what to expect. What happens when you fast is that toxins and waste products begin to pour from the system at a very rapid rate. In fact, depending on your previous lifestyle, the symptoms are not dissimilar to those of drug withdrawal at times. Also, these symptoms may be experienced in a milder form when you change your diet to any of the options in the Perfect Health program.

Many people experience unpleasant symptoms when they make the change to a more natural diet. Some people traipse off to the doctor, who then informs them that they have either a virus or that this diet does not suit them. Then, an antibiotic is prescribed, even though there is nothing an antibiotic can do to a virus.

It is unreasonable to assume that you can put garbage into your body for years and then not experience some unpleasant symptoms as your body repairs itself. The worse your past diet and the more medication (including headache tablets and painkillers) you have been on the worse your symptoms can be.

The most common symptoms from just a change in diet are cold- and flu-like symptoms—headaches, excess mucus, sore throat, nasal congestion, etc. It is best in this case (or with any other symptoms) to get into bed, sleep as much as possible, and drink plenty of filtered water and freshly extracted fruit and vegetable juices. The next most common symptom is an upset stomach and/or constipation. Both these symptoms are a result of old fecal matter being encouraged to leave the digestive tract, by either expelling this old matter very rapidly or, with constipation, the old matter forms a plug. In this case a saline solution enema used first thing each morning for two to three days would help clear the path and you should be on your way to comfortable bowel movements.

Other symptoms of detoxification can range from headaches (which could last up to one week, especially if you have been drinking or eating foods that contain caffeine), irritability, nausea, violent vomiting, insomnia, extreme coldness, temperature or fever, copious expulsion of mucus from almost any bodily orifice (from the nose to the vagina—but don't panic, it's not an infection!), bad breath, coated tongue, weakness, tiredness, muscular aches and pains, dizziness, and heart palpitations even when lying down (this is simply the body dealing with a stimulant that may have been lurking for years).

In fact, one of the interesting things about a period of detoxification is that the body retraces past problems, so you may find an old injury flaring up, or your mouth may taste of vitamins or medication that you may have taken some time previously. One of the most fascinating detox stories I have ever encountered was about a man who tasted sulfur in his mouth forty years after having taken sulfur medication. His urine also smelled very strongly of sulfur for a while during his fast.

The reason for this is that the body often *wraps* a harmful substance or waste product in fat and stores it until it has the time and energy to deal with it. Making a habit of eating poorly combined, highly processed meals and the regular use of medication, alcohol, and cigarettes leads to levels of toxicity that the body cannot effectively deal with while you sleep (remember that most of the body's repair work happens at this time). So, slowly over the years, these poisons accumulate in the tissues and conditions like cancer may eventually arise, causing damage to surrounding cells and tissues. Fasting and cleansing diets are the best way to break down these toxic stores and eliminate them from the body.

Try as best as you can to avoid medical intervention. If, for example, you are suffering from caffeine withdrawal and your head is pounding so badly that you cannot function, it would be better to drink half a cup of coffee or even a full one at that, than take a painkiller. Then maybe reduce the caffeine slowly by blending half-decaffeinated coffee with your regular coffee for a few weeks or a month, and then further by blending two-thirds decaffeinated coffee and then up to three-quarters until you can stop completely without feeling awful!

Don't for a moment think that you will only experience these unpleasant symptoms once. The body will simply not dump all the old waste matter and toxins into your bloodstream at one time; it will do so little by little as it gets stronger and better able to cope. The whole process of repairing your body takes at least two years, and during these two years (or more) you will experience various healing crises. In these instances heed the good old-fashioned advice to drink plenty of fluids (filtered or spring water first or freshly extracted fruit and vegetable juices), go to bed, and get plenty of rest. Within twenty-four to forty-eight hours most symptoms will be gone and you will feel wonderful!

If you are unable to go to bed and have to be at work, I suggest you eat only raw, uncooked, fresh fruit and vegetables, juices, and raw nuts and seeds and try and pace yourself, making sure you at least get to bed early. I have found many people take a few heaped teaspoons of dried barley grass powder when they feel any detox symptoms coming on, get into bed, and in the morning they are fine.

Whatever you do, take things easy and slowly and rest as much as possible.

FAY'S STORY

I grew up as a little girl on a farm and knew little of candy and junk food. We thrived on fruit that we picked straight from the trees after having to climb them first. Our vegetables were homegrown in a big vegetable patch in our backyard. We had milk, cream, and butter from my dad's own small dairy herd that did not get added hormones, antibiotics, or lot feeding in those days. We also had a chicken run with fowls, which were slaughtered, plucked, and dressed for the table in the backyard. Yuck! My dad hunted for wild fowl and buck, so venison was on the table, too. We lived a simple, carefree life for the first part of my young life. When I reached high school we moved to the city, which was a huge culture shock for us. Of course we did get introduced to junk food and a not-so-healthy lifestyle. Looking back, however, as I grew up I recall always making an effort to eat healthy with the limited knowledge that I had.

By the time I married, I was rather "health-conscious" and made every effort to feed my family as healthy as possible and made an endeavor to eliminate dead foods, but knew little of true healthy eating. At least I knew about avoiding additives, preservatives, margarine, refined foods, etc., and making sure that I read all labels. I was introduced to Mary-Ann Shearer's book *The Natural Way*. I was delighted, as this was so much easier to follow. I was only partially converted at that time, as I would never have given up animal products. It just wasn't the done thing. You had to have meat and dairy to get your protein—or so I thought.

Strangely as the years went by, my body began to tell me it did not want meat. I would feel a strange heaviness in my stomach after eating meat, especially red meat or pork. So I cut back to only eating chicken or fish in small portions, which made me feel a bit better. I continued to follow Mary-Ann's advice on and off from then on.

In 1995 I was going through a difficult time and landed in the hospital for two weeks on sleep therapy due to an emotional breakdown. I was consequently put on heavy medication, i.e., sleeping tablets, antidepressants, and anti-anxiety tablets. I weaned myself off after about two years as I could not bear the zombie-like feeling of not belonging to myself.

During this time my therapist felt I needed to see an endocrinologist as she felt my hormones were out of balance. I was referred to this specialist who diagnosed me as having gone into early menopause and informed me that my ovaries were shriveled; he said that blood tests showed that I had very low estrogen levels—I was thirty-nine years old.

Here is the concoction he put me on, which nearly killed me:

Treatment No 1 6/8/97
ABDOMINAL Hormone implant under the skin
3 x 20mg oestradiol implant - pellets
1 x 25mg testosterone implant - pellets
1 x Estring [inserted over cervix] (later removed as it caused vaginal irritation)
ORAL - daily dose
Premarin .625 x 1 at night D 1-26 increased to 1.25mg and further increased to 2.5mg [over 17mths]
Provera 5mg ½ tab at night from D13
Nootropil 400mg cap 1 x 3 a day
Caltrate 300mg x 3 at night
Vitrace cap x 1 a day
Testosterone increased to 25mg x 2
Oestradiol increased to 20mg x 5 then later down to 4 toward the end.

At first I felt good on these treatments, but as the months went by I began to feel worse than when I started.

I began to have severe bleeds. The bad bleeding started at the end of August 1998. Blood suddenly dripped as if from a tap into the toilet bowl when I went to the bathroom. I got a huge fright. I was away from home and had to go to another doctor. This doctor was shocked at the treatment I was receiving and strongly urged me to stop, as he believed I was high at risk for developing cancer with these "massive" doses of hormones. I was taken aback. I trusted this specialist! However, after much thought I made my decision and began weaning myself off the oral medication at the end of 1998.

The next severe bleed was in April 1999. I saturated about twenty-five sanitary towels in one day. As the saying goes, I bled like a pig. The bleeding would not stop so I just stood in the bath; large clots that fit in the palm of my hand just dropped out of me and splattered into the tub. It looked like a slaughter house. I would just stand there and cry.

I had more than ten severe bleeds from then on. Some days were very heavy, leaving me quite weak and washed out. Other days were medium to light.

From December 5, 2000, to February 7, 2001, I began bleeding continuously (I did not have a day without bleeding). This was the first time that the bleeding had gone on for so long at one stretch.

I reluctantly went to my GP for a consultation. He immediately asked when to book me in for surgery and said I needed a blood transfusion, but decided to give me an iron infusion instead. I later went into hypothermia and had a horrid reaction after the drip. I had terrible cold shivers that I could not control; a hot water bottle wasn't enough and my husband and son eventually had to carry me and get me into a hot bath to warm me up. I was also awfully nauseated and all my muscles were terribly sore and weak. I could not eat or even sit up. I crawled into bed with the electric blanket on high all night to keep warm and eventually fell asleep. I felt a little better in the morning.

My hair started falling out quite badly; in fact I hardly had any left. My ponytail was thinner than my baby finger. It fell out evenly, not in chunks—no bald patches. (I have always had fairly thin hair, but this was different—it had never been this bad.) I combed out a lot daily and I'd also see lots floating in the bath after washing it.

I had discomfort and at times pain in my finger joints. I had a stiff and sore lower back—lower lumbar spine and sacrum. I had a stiff neck, especially the right side into the muscle, swelling of hands and feet from time to time, and a bloated tummy. My general vision deteriorated rapidly and got worse for close-up work. I could not see without using glasses or a magnifying glass. My fingernails and toenails had thick ridges. I had nasty headaches that developed into migraines, my skin started to go yellow, and I was losing weight.

Early in 1999 I had gone on a detox program, as per the Natural Way. I was doing well for a good while and I felt wonderful—everyone commented on how great and young I looked. For various reasons I took a wobble and went back to my old habits for a bit and felt awful.

At this point I did not know which way to turn; I contacted Mary-Ann on July 7, 2001, for help as I was feeling desperate and needed some serious help. After a careful assessment of my diet and many questions, she put me on Perfect Health, removing all animal products because of the hormone levels in the animal products that would trigger my problem. I also went on Barley Life juice, beetroot/pineapple juice, and flaxseed oil. Within thirty-six hours the bleeding totally stopped. It was amazing. I was thrilled. Needless to say, I was converted. I was prepared to stick with this as I was determined to keep my uterus and not go on any medication again.

I was diligent and very strict with my way of eating and did not cheat at all. I so wanted to get completely better. However, a few months later I felt that my health began to deteriorate. I started to get other symptoms: sores in my mouth, very yellow skin tone, vaginal irritation, no energy, battles for breath, heart palpitations, nausea, weakness, dizziness, a fuzzy head, and I was also very weepy and emotional.

After I had contacted Mary-Ann again, she asked me to have a blood test done for my iron levels. This I did and sent her the results:

Serum Iron	2.9 [l]
Transferrin	48.2 [h]
Iron Saturation	3.0 [l]
Ferritin	2.6 [l]

Mary-Ann also recommended that I see a doctor whom she trusted as she said the heavy blood loss over such an extended period had resulted in severe anemia. The doctor offered a "nature cure." This doctor was truly unique in that he was the first ever to give me a caring three-hour consultation, thoroughly examining me and asking every possible question regarding my condition; after which his only prescription was a two-week stay at the hydro with a supervised fast. My husband was of course horrified as he felt I was too weak, had lost weight, and that I was in no condition to be put on a fast. But I was willing to do whatever the doctor asked; I just wanted to get better without having to resort to surgery and have my uterus removed.

The doctor felt that over many years, damage could have accumulated to a potentially irreversible level. He hoped this not to be the case, and that we should keep an open mind. He said our aim was ultimately a "nature cure." But bearing in mind my previous lifestyle and its influence over many years, it was conceivable that my uterus was not salvageable. We were also to bear in mind that life is too preciously short to waste years on resolving a problem that could perhaps not be solved anyway. He suggested that I should make peace with the idea that I could end up with a hysterectomy, even if it only confirmed our own inability to solve the problems correctly. He would try his best to conserve me "intact" as was my wish. He suggested we give it a good chance, exploiting every tool available, and only if they failed to consider resorting to the surgical alternative. He was, however, legally, ethically, and morally bound not to promise me success and advised me along the orthodox route if all evidence pointed that way. The doctor also said, "So following Mary-Ann's advice did better than all the hormones and drugs, it seems!" YES, IT CERTAINLY DID!!

I was booked in for a supervised fast with hydrotherapy to assist with the elimination of toxins. This was not easy as I was extremely weak. At times they were not able to read my blood sugar or my blood pressure. The doctor said that a two-week fast was ideal but he had no expectations of me lasting that long; he would be satisfied if I could manage up to three days, taking one day at a time. Well, I managed four and a half days. There were times when I really thought I could not do it anymore. But I worked hard at speaking to myself and reminding myself that this was for my health, my future, and my family. When you are not well, you truly value and long for good health. After the fast I was slowly introduced to papaya juice and gradually on to Perfect Health, which I stuck to very strictly according to Mary-Ann's instructions.

This is my testimony in a letter to Mary-Ann after the supervised fast:

Hi Mary-Ann,

Home at last and happy to be with my family; I can't explain to you how much better I am feeling. As you said earlier, you were confident God was going to use this time to repair my body, and He most certainly did. I am forever grateful to Him, you, and the doctor. Well, so is my family. Everyone says how my color has improved; my boys say I am chirpier—overall, a great improvement. My energy levels are up—I feel much stronger (still a way to go), my appetite is also good, and I managed to pick up some weight, so I'm not looking gaunt. My brain is not so foggy—I can hold a normal conversation without so much brain freeze. No more vaginal irritation or bleed-

ing. No more breathlessness and thighs not so weak. Not as weepy or as cold, etc. The last three days at the hydro I went on some good walks and felt as though I could run up the mountain (which I didn't of course). I felt as though I could fly; I don't know if you know what I mean. I felt full of life and had a spring in my step. On Monday, the doctor said he was amazed at my improvement and that he saw a first genuine smile. He also mentioned that I had him worried as he had only given me a fifty/fifty chance, as he had never seen a case like this with such low blood sugar levels—he said I survived on ketones for five days—and they're what kept me going while on the fast. As you said, I was a walking miracle! Who would normally believe that fasting, hydrotherapy, and prayer could have such a positive impact on the human body in such a short space of time? Our God is truly a powerful and merciful Father. I trust Him that I am going to get stronger each day.

I am fasting today as the doctor has instructed (for thirty-six hours once a week) and will also continue with Perfect Health, with no animal products as per your advice of which he fully agrees with. I will also continue with the barley grass juice, flaxseed oil, and beet juice. The doctor says I may still have some bleeding episodes and that they will hopefully get less and less. The desire of my heart is still NOT to have a hysterectomy, although I do understand what he says about having quality of life without a uterus rather than a miserable life with a uterus. He suggests we give it six months or so with the nature cure approach. My iron levels have already improved dramatically.

Sincerely with all my heart.

Love, Fay

UPDATE: FIVE YEARS LATER

I'm happy to report that I turned fifty in December 2006 and am feeling great. I still follow Perfect Health, as does my whole family now and we have better health than when we were younger. My hemoglobin levels have continued to rise and have been at a consistent level of 13.1 since December 19, 2002, and all the other blood levels are in the normal range. I am so blessed!!

RECAP

- Fasting is a wonderfully quick and efficient way to regain health, lose weight, and give your body a rest
- However, unpleasant symptoms may occur and these can be frightening if you are not being supervised or have not prepared yourself beforehand by reading as much information as possible on the subject
- It is also vital to start and break a fast correctly and only a trained supervisor can help you with this
- Detoxification is part of the healing process, so hang in there—it too will pass and your health will improve dramatically

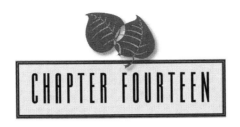

CHAPTER FOURTEEN

Weight Loss and Weight Gain
The Secret

I COME FROM A FAMILY where most of the women (on both sides of my family) are overweight. As much as I strived to be tall and willowy, I had to be content with curves in all the wrong places.

I think part of my passion for health when I was younger was a fear of being obese, so I exercised and tried to do the right thing and my weight would fluctuate within a 20-pound range. I remember so clearly that when I finally felt I was thin enough I was actually underweight but more than that I was at my sickest. I had just been told I had a chemical imbalance of the brain and would have to live on medication for life; I then developed allergies and began to suffer from allergic dermatitis and rhinitis. I took vitamin supplements; I made my own yogurt, muesli, and whole wheat bread; nothing changed. I changed the brand of supplements and still nothing changed. I remember so clearly one morning in desperation I cried out to God and asked Him please to give me wisdom and show me where I was going wrong. Within days, I believe He did and the Natural Way is the result. Now for more than twenty years I have not had a doctor's bill because of ill health (neither has my family) and my weight has been stable at a level that is right for my bone structure and genetics. It was only when I started focusing on my health that my weight was finally sorted out. When I started looking at the nutritional value of foods and stopped looking at the energy (kilojoule or calorie) value my life and body turned around. I would wake up with loads of energy, my stomach worked, my allergies cleared up, and my brain chemistry was balanced, and as the months passed my weight stabilized at the correct level and has stayed there for nearly twenty years.

The secret to managing my weight was twofold:

1. I had to focus on getting healthy.
2. I had to learn to listen to my body.

Both of these steps took some time to implement as I had to re-educate myself. For example, I had always tried to keep fats out of my diet, but now I understand that without the right fats (see chapter eight) my hormonal system would not work properly and that is the very system that controls body weight and appetite.

I learned that refined sugar, instead of "giving me go," actually made me tired and encouraged my body to store fat as it resulted in low blood sugar, which tends to have that effect.

I found that fresh fruit was more nutritious than diet cereals, and that artificial sweeteners and diet sodas could actually slow down my metabolism and increase my appetite, contributing to weight problems. It was one huge learning curve and the results have been exceptional.

Then I had to listen to my body. This was a huge issue as I was a compulsive overeater; I was permanently hungry. I could feel completely stuffed and at the same time be ravenously hungry. I learned that when your cells are not getting the right nutrients they keep sending a message to the brain screaming for the right stuff. Now it would be wonderful if every morning you woke up with a printout hanging out of your mouth telling you exactly what to eat, but in the real world you wake up and grab the nearest thing and rush off to work and hope for the best. In chapter three I cover listening to your body in great detail so flip back if you need a refresher. What I find works is to acknowledge that we have God-made bodies and that we need to feed these bodies God-made food, which will result in God-made health. If we insist on eating man-made food we will suffer from man-made diseases such as obesity and weight issues (to name but a few).

There are other factors involved, such as a metabolism ruined by going on too many fad or crash diets. These only encourage your body to store fuel more effectively and efficiently so as to be ready for the next time you starve yourself. Fasting correctly, by the way, does not have this effect.

Another reason often given for a weight problem is a hormonal imbalance or a glandular problem. This is often used as an excuse for bad living habits. Many people who have this problem are often extremely undisciplined in their eating habits and frequently eat late at night. If a hormonal problem truly exists (blood tests would confirm this), it can be sorted out in the long term by eating correctly, getting healthy, and listening to your body. For example, refined sugar in your diet can affect your blood sugar level, and this in turn can affect the function of the pituitary gland, the adrenal glands, and the thyroid gland. Just by eliminating refined sugar from the diet, these glands can return to normal function. Changing to an artificial sweetener is no better as it interferes with the endocrine system just as much, if not more, so instead sweeten with raw honey or fructose powder (in small quantities).

Caffeine and vinegar are two stimulants used in diet products that can both affect the thyroid gland. When an organ or gland is continually stimulated artificially (as in this case) its activity can become depressed. In other words, from continual stimulation, the thyroid gland can slow down and not function as efficiently as it should. This could result in a sluggish metabolism and difficulty in losing weight. Remember that vinegar is a by-product of fermentation in the stomach, yet another reason to combine your food properly. If you need a sour taste, a much healthier choice is fresh lemon juice or small quantities of apple, grape, or Balsamic vinegar (just check the label for sulfur dioxide). Mustard oil, found in garlic and onions, can also affect the thyroid gland. Mustard oil can, through a series of events, suppress the production of the hormone thyroxin, which is the hormone that regulates the rate at which we burn fuel. By cutting these substances out of the diet those affected organs and glands will eventually function correctly. I have found that this can take from two months to two years, or longer. A supervised fast can correct the endocrine glands very quickly (see chapter thirteen), or try a period on completely raw food only (two to six weeks would be ideal).

Gluten (the protein found only in grain and products made from grain, such as wheat, rye, oats, and barley) has now been shown to interfere with endocrine (hormonal) function. I have found that if I eat even one slice of organic whole wheat bread, for five days in a row, I can gain 5 pounds in weight. That is because I am gluten intolerant. If you want to see the effect of not eating gluten on your body, remove all gluten-containing foods for at least six weeks because that is how long it takes to see an improvement. So often people remove gluten for a week and see no improvement and go back to eating these foods. In time when you eat these foods every few weeks you may have no response, but if you eat them for more than three or more days you usually do. One of the advantages of removing gluten from your diet is that your skin and bowel functions improve dramatically.

Another reason for a persistent weight problem could be that you are on some type of medication—anything from contraceptive pills to thyroid drugs, or even plain old headache tablets or laxatives could be the culprits. Any drug can wreak havoc on your body and I suggest that with the help of a good doctor, you wean yourself off all medication. To achieve this, you would start by taking a smaller dose; that is, if you were taking ten units of medication, you would start by reducing your intake to five units. You would then progress to taking it every second day, then every third day, and so on until you were able to limit your intake to once a week. Finally you will be able to stop altogether. It is vital that you consult a doctor before attempting to wean yourself off any medication. Just make sure you are speaking to a doctor who is aware and supportive of a natural lifestyle, who would like to see you well and drug-free.

Often it is difficult to know where to start in order to achieve a slimmer, healthier body. Many people have asked me for a diet sheet as a guide to how much to eat and how often. I have always been reluctant to do this as the Perfect Health program is not so much a diet as a lifestyle and you must learn to listen to your body and its own particular needs. But I have since come to realize that for many dieters who have followed a regime that requires everything to be weighed and measured, to change over to a lifestyle that allows them to eat as much as they like is like giving an alcoholic the key to a liquor store. As a result, I've put together various flexible programs that make the transition easier. What you have to decide is which program suits you best. That way you are making the final decision and are not left feeling totally restricted. If you need a more detailed program with recipes and day-to-day guidance, go to www.mary-anns.com and join our "100 days to health" program.

Before you start, remember that this is a lifestyle, not a religion! You can adapt your meals within the Perfect Health principles. There will be times when you will fail to stick to the program. Do not become disheartened; instead follow the guidelines in this chapter to help you get over those times and prevent them from recurring too often. Take note—I said "too often," not "ever again." Don't be unrealistic; we live in a world filled with an endless variety of junk food that is packaged, designed, and promoted in such a way to get us drooling. We have restaurants and fast-food outlets on every corner, just begging us to come in and celebrate something. But do not despair. You will be able to resist temptation if you stick to a few simple basics:

1. Do your best to combine your food correctly. If you can't, skipping the next meal often does wonders to sort out the mess in your stomach. But don't do this too often as you will merely be taking one step forward and two steps back. If you are still hungry after a badly combined meal, then stick to neutral salads and vegetables (see the food-combining chart on page 265 and the recipe section in chapter eighteen).

2. Do not feel guilty if you break the rules. You'll be paying enough of a price physically so don't make it worse by punishing yourself mentally, as well. Guilt can often cause you to go on a rebellious binge, which will cause even more damage both mentally and physically.

3. Do not stock "no-no's" anywhere in your home. If ice cream, cakes, cookies, and chocolates are bad for you, they are equally bad for your family. It is not a sign of good housekeeping to always have a tub of ice cream in the freezer or a stock of cookies in a jar. It is simply a bad habit. No matter how strong-willed you think you are, you will want to eat these snacks just because they are there. Even I would!

4. Do, at all times, stock a large variety of the good things and let them be on display. You know what it's like when all that's in the house is a couple of bananas and one or two apples—boring, boring, boring. Who would possibly feel like fruit? But imagine a couple of strategically placed bowls or baskets filled to overflowing with nectarines, pineapples, mangoes, strawberries, kiwi, grapes, plums, and peaches, and perhaps even a bowl or two of dates, raisins, or nuts. Who could possibly resist?

5. Remember that presentation is almost as important as taste. If food doesn't look good, you won't feel like eating it. Concentrate on making the good food look even better. With very little effort a fresh fruit salad with cashew cream (see recipe section) can look far more enticing than a donut.

6. Always start all cooked meals with raw vegetables or a salad.

7. Eat an entire meal each day that consists of fresh fruit—you can include preservative-free dried fruit or raw nuts or seeds with this meal.

8. Snack on fresh or preservative-free dried fruit before you eat processed candy and snack on avocado, raw nuts, olives, or a salad with extra-virgin vegetable oil before you eat fries, chips, or other processed or animal fats such as cheese and pizza.

9. Make sure you eat animal protein no more than once a day and no bigger a portion than the size and thickness of the palm of your hand.

10. Try and eat starches such as potatoes or rice not more than once a day unless you are trying to gain weight, and keep the daily quantity to an amount that would fit in one cupped hand.

11. Drink a glass of water before you eat anything, even a snack. You may be confusing the signal for thirst with hunger.

12. Don't weigh yourself unless you like being depressed. Rather, try on a pair of pants or a skirt once a week if you really want to see how you are doing.

13. Don't weigh or measure your fresh fruit and vegetables; you may eat as much as you like!

Below are three basic options based on the Perfect Health program, to help you establish good healthy eating habits. You must decide which of the three you feel most comfortable with and which one enables you to maintain your weight at the right level.

Option 1

WAKE-UP

Glass of one of the following: water or hot water with fresh lemon, freshly squeezed fruit juice, or barley grass juice with flaxseed oil.

BREAKFAST

Half a large papaya filled with a sliced banana and half a cup of chopped dates. Or one banana, one apple, and one pear, diced together and sprinkled with half a cup of raisins. Or any three fruits from the sweet and sub-acid columns (see chart at the back of the book) with a quarter to half a cup of dates or raisins. (Or swap with Option 2 breakfast.)

MID-MORNING (BETWEEN 10 A.M. AND NOON)

Try any one of the following options:

1 whole pineapple
2 oranges
3 tangerines
2 mangoes
5 kiwi
2 apples
3–4 peaches
1 large bunch of grapes
8 litchis
8 strawberries
6 apricots
2 pears
1–2 papaya
As much watermelon or other melon as you like

Mid-morning and breakfast may be swapped; just make sure you are getting a good variety of fruit. No tea or coffee should be drunk during the morning. (The caffeine will affect your kidneys, and you will end up retaining water and your endocrine system will possibly slow your metabolism.) Drink only water, either hot or cold. Fresh fruit juice may also be drunk, only if you are thirsty—and try diluting it fifty/fifty with water.

LUNCH

Make a very large salad with any of the following ingredients: lettuce, tomato, celery, red pepper, carrot, spinach, sprouts, cabbage, broccoli, cauliflower, grated butternut squash, zucchini, mushrooms, green beans, or any other raw vegetable. Half an avocado may be added to this or used in the following dressing: blend together half an avocado, a little celery, a strip of red pepper, herbal salt, and a tomato. Add some water or fresh lemon juice if it is too thick. This salad may be eaten on its own or, if you are very hungry, with one of the following (also see recipe section):

   1 large baked potato
   2 corn on the cob
   1 medium bowl of brown rice
   2 slices homemade whole wheat bread
   3 slices 100 percent rye
   4 whole wheat, rice, or corn crackers
   1 whole wheat pita bread

MID-AFTERNOON (3 P.M.–5 P.M.)

A portion of any one type of fruit, such as an apple, orange, two peaches, or whatever fits into your loosely cupped hands.

DINNER

Dinner must be started with a large side plate of fresh salad followed with as many steamed vegetables as you like. You may add any of the starches mentioned for lunch if all you had for lunch was the salad. Alternatively, you may like to add half a cup of unsalted, unroasted nuts, or a portion of oven-grilled fish or organic chicken. For a more tasty option, place the chicken or fish in a casserole dish with mushrooms, celery, red pepper, or any vegetable of your choice, adding herbal salt and a selection of herbs and bake in a hot oven until done.

Lunch and dinner may be switched, but remember not to have either starch or protein more than once a day. In other words, if you have a potato for lunch, you should not have rice for supper, and if you had nuts for lunch you should not have fish for supper. Try not to eat after 8 P.M. but if you need to snack after supper, any raw vegetable is suitable.

You may find you sleep better after eating starches in the evening as they help raise your serotonin levels. Protein for lunch also helps keep you awake as it tends to have a stimulatory effect on the brain.

Option 2

This is the way my family eats. It is a lot easier than Option 1, not only in preparation but also when it comes to listening to your body.

WAKE-UP

A glass of water (preferably filtered) with two teaspoons powdered barley grass juice with one tablespoon organic cold-pressed flaxseed oil or blend.

BREAKFAST

A glass of freshly squeezed juice, usually orange as it is the most convenient to extract. In my family, most of us are usually not particularly hungry until about 10 A.M. and since we now listen to our bodies, we don't eat much until then. We find it convenient to eat nuts at breakfast-time. We tend to stick to almonds or cashews but also enjoy Brazil nuts and pecans and eat a quarter to half a cup each with our acid fruit. What we love best is our nut shake or smoothie (see recipe section).

MID-MORNING

One to three pieces of any fruit (properly combined). Most often we will eat just one type of fruit at a time, such as one to two oranges or apples, or just a large bunch of grapes, or one to two mangoes. On the days where we eat nuts for breakfast, we are not particularly hungry during the morning. It is best to stick to acid or sub-acid fruits for at least four hours after a nut meal.

LUNCH

We then get hungry again between noon and 2 P.M. and eat two bananas and a handful of dates or raisins, for example. We might have a pineapple or half a papaya or whatever is in season and delicious.

If you prefer, have a large fresh salad with some steamed or grilled vegetables. Vegetables are likely to speed up weight loss as they (especially salad vegetables) use up more energy in the process of digestion than they give to the body.

MID-AFTERNOON

At about 3 to 5 P.M. we might feel like snacking and have a piece of fruit or half a cup of preservative-free dried fruit such as dates or raisins.

DINNER

Occasionally this is also fruit, especially in summer when there aren't enough hours in the day to eat all the delicious fruits available. Most often, though, we'll start with a large salad consisting of lettuce, tomato, carrots, red pepper, celery, avocado, and occasionally some olives (in brine). Some evenings we make a complete meal of this and others we might have whole baked butternut squash, steamed broccoli, baked or steamed potatoes, bowls of steaming brown rice, steamed corn on the cob, a mixed vegetable casserole, or soup. (See recipe section and our Web site.) We do put a bit of butter on our cooked food, although I do find that if I'm eating avocado, I do not need the butter. I find olive oil far more palatable than butter, and as it is cold-pressed, unsaturated, and cholesterol-free, it is a far healthier choice (it is less fattening, too!). If avocado is not freely available, especially in summer, we might have a meal of just salad and half a cup of nuts each. Remember that if you are a vegetarian, a quarter to half a cup of nuts or seeds should be included in your diet at least three times a week.

Option 3

This is a cleansing diet and although it is very healthy and efficient in helping you reach your ideal weight, it is quite difficult to maintain for more than a couple of weeks at a time due to the fact that it is a totally raw food diet. I would encourage everyone, young, old, fat, thin, sick, or healthy to try this at least once a year for a two-week period.

Your day is very similar to that outlined in Option 2 in that you eat fruit all day, whenever you feel hungry. Supper could either be more fruit, or alternatively a large salad with half a cup of unsalted, unroasted nuts or an avocado. The salad with nuts or avocado should be eaten at least three to four times a week, but you will find it easier to stick to this program if you have a quarter to half a cup of nuts or seeds a day. If you are not wanting to lose weight on this raw food regime, then make sure to eat more avocados, dates, and raisins, as well as try to eat at least two bananas a day.

With all the programs outlined in this chapter, the most important thing of all is to listen to your body, not to your taste buds, and to remember that this can take a couple of months to achieve. Also, do not overeat! I cannot reiterate this often enough. Eat slowly, chew carefully, and keep it simple; the simpler the meal, the less done and added to the food, the better. Simple meals are more often far more attractive and tastier than complicated ones, and a great deal more healthy, too!

You may find it difficult to stick to your newly chosen eating program and the sudden introduction of regular exercise into your lifestyle may cause some discomfort. Refer to the ten points listed below from time to time to help you keep on track.

Check-List for Weight Loss

1. Am I Exercising Aerobically at Least Five Times per Week for a Minimum Period of Thirty Minutes (Walking Briskly, Swimming, Running, or Cycling)?

Exercises such as stretching, tennis, gardening, and other stop/start activities should not be counted in this thirty-minute period, but should be regarded as additional exercise. Remember to start slowly and to build up your time gradually—start with five minutes per day, then build up to ten minutes and then fifteen minutes until you eventually reach thirty minutes per day. Regular daily exercise, even for only a few minutes, is more preferable than starting with thirty minutes of exercise three times a week.

2. Am I off All Possible Medication?

If not, remember to work toward this with the help of a good doctor, one who knows that all drugs are a strain on the body.

3. Am I Following the Most Basic Guidelines of the Perfect Health Program?

These are:

- Fruit in the morning with nuts
- A salad or raw vegetables with each meal
- Correctly combined meals
- Preferably animal protein no more than once a day
- No dairy products, tea, or coffee, or at least reduce intake each week little by little

- No additives in any foods
- Animal fats such as butter and cream no more than once a day
- Eat in moderation, and only when hungry
- Do not eat after sunset as the digestive tract slows down after the sun has set. Try at least not to eat after 8 P.M. if you can or if you do, keep the meal very light and stick to just neutral vegetables or fresh fruit
- Remove all refined sugar and carbohydrates

4. Am I Doing Something to Renew My Mind?

For example, read some motivational material on a regular basis. Any bookshop will be able to help you find some stimulating reading matter. I find the Bible the most inspiring. Other books I have enjoyed are *The Purpose-Driven Life* (Rick Warren), *Man's Search for Meaning* (Victor Frankl), *How to Stop Worrying and Start Living* (Dale Carnegie), *Failing Forward* (John Maxwell), and *Wild at Heart* (John Eldridge).

5. Am I Developing Interests That Do Not Focus on Me or My Weight?

Go to art lessons, help out at your local school or church, or join a help organization such as Lifeline. I've found that people who have a real emotional problem with food are usually too busy thinking about themselves, their bodies, and what goes into them! By doing something that involves helping other people or by learning something new, you take the focus off yourself, and suddenly what you put into your mouth is not of such obsessive interest any more.

I remember doing the Dale Carnegie Course in 1983. It was a turning point in my life. Mark and I did the course on human relations and public speaking together. By doing the course, I learned to accept myself, and not to be so critical and judgmental of myself and others. I became more tolerant as a result and stopped feeling guilty about not being Miss Perfect. I started focusing on small successes instead of what I had perceived as huge failures. I think women in particular are too obsessed with an unrealistic image of perfection that we strive toward, and then we suffer from tremendous guilt because we haven't attained our impossible goal. Relax and be positive about yourself for a change.

Learn to love yourself; it is vital in order to be able to love your neighbor and it is not about your ego.

6. Have I Identified any Trigger Events That Cause Me to Eat Badly?

A trigger event could be an emotion such as happiness, sadness, anger, or frustration that makes you want to eat everything in sight. Once you have identified it, you will be able to do something about it when the urge to indulge crops up.

Ask God to help you let go of this baggage, as often we battle to do this on our own.

7. Am I Still Eating Too Much?

Eating too much is when you get up from the table feeling "as full as a tick." Also remember to check your fat intake. Do not eat more than one type of fat per day if you are overweight. Remember, the more natural a fat, the better it is for you—avocados and nuts are a better source of fat than butter, but butter is a better source of fat than margarine. Do not exclude natural fats from your diet altogether, as they contain the essential fatty acids that help your metabolic rate and hormonal system function properly. Diets that prohibit natural fats are dangerous.

8. Can I See Myself Slim?

Lie in bed each night before going to sleep, and see the new, slim you. Visualize yourself with more energy and eating only healthy foods. It's vitally important for the successful attainment of your goal weight to be able to see yourself as you want to be.

9. Don't Ever Compare Myself with Other People

You are unique and one-of-a-kind. Your bone structure is unique, your metabolism is unique, and so are your genes. Be a better you...not like someone else.

10. If I Am Eating When Bored, Sad, Depressed, or to Fill an Emptiness Inside, Remember That Only God Can Fill That Void.

Begin by asking Him to reveal His love for you and His purpose for your life. *The Purpose-Driven Life* by Rick Warren will get you on track within forty days. I, too, ate in this frame of mind so I speak from experience. Making healthier choices when it came to food helped my relationship with God and this in turn is what satisfied me.

Remember, if you have abused your body by going on and off various diets, it will take a while to rectify your metabolism. In the meantime, exercise regularly, start your day with some fruit, include raw vegetables with all meals other than fruit meals, combine your food correctly, and start to renew your mind by reading and learning more about your health. Banish all refined foods, sweeteners, and additives from your diet. Keep yourself busy. But most importantly, remember that the Perfect Health program is not a diet or a religion; it is a lifestyle and it takes time to alter the habits of a lifetime.

What about Gaining Weight?

If your problem is the opposite, that is if you are too thin and cannot gain weight, it is often a lot more difficult to correct. People with a slender build are usually genetically predisposed to thinness and are unlikely to become well-rounded.

But all is not lost—there are several steps you can take to pad yourself out a little. However, a few things need to be clarified first.

A change to the Perfect Health program usually results in weight loss, and this applies equally to those who are overweight at the onset and those who are underweight. This is the result of your body working through a catabolic phase, which is a breaking down of unhealthy tissue. This process could take anywhere from two weeks to a year before the metabolism stabilizes and no further weight is lost. You may find this unwanted weight loss frustrating, particularly if you have increased your food intake in order to gain weight. But eating huge quantities at every meal during the catabolic phase could, ironically, cause further weight loss. The body is placed under unnecessary strain and cannot break the food down efficiently, resulting in poor absorption of nutrients. It would be better to eat smaller portions more frequently.

As always, listen to your body. Concentrate on increasing the proportion of high-energy food in your diet—avocados, dates (and all other dried fruits), bananas, and natural unprocessed starches such as potatoes, brown rice, and corn on the cob are all suitable. By eating small portions of high-energy food more often, you will find that you will experience a gradual weight gain. Also, increase the quantity of fruit in your diet. Try eating less salad—salad is a negative-energy food as it requires more energy from the body for digestion than it in fact gives to the body after digestion. By adding some cold-pressed oil to your salads you will increase their energy value significantly.

After the stabilization phase, which could last up to a year, your body will go through a rebuilding or anabolic phase. However, you will only experience this when your body is ready; it cannot be rushed along. Fasting under strict supervision is the only way to speed up the process of catabolism, stabilization, and anabolism and many underweight people actually correct their metabolism by fasting under supervision.

Weight training or resistance exercise done under the guidance of a qualified instructor can help build your body in all the right places. However, you do need to be diligent about your training and keep it up until you see results.

You may also find that the very foods that cause people to gain weight may be the ones causing you to lose weight. Caffeine can speed up your metabolism as can artificial sweeteners (remember that if you are overweight it can slow down your metabolism). Gluten is known to cause weight loss in people suffering from celiac disease, which is a form of gluten intolerance, and weight gain in those with a tendency to be overweight.

If you still battle to gain weight after following these suggestions, console yourself with the fact that thinner people generally age slower and live a longer, healthier life and experience less strain on joints and organs.

Remember to focus on getting well and staying healthy and try not to be distracted by either weight gain or weight loss. In time your body will function at its optimum level, regardless of whether you have a sleek or a nicely rounded shape. Your ultimate reward will be glowing health, loads of energy, and peace of mind.

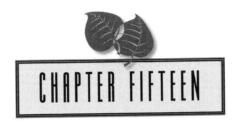

CHAPTER FIFTEEN

A Husband's Perspective
Mark Shearer

AS FAR BACK as I can remember, I have enjoyed eating, and for my sins, I ended up in the restaurant business, as well. With this thought in mind, let me tell you why I am writing a chapter in this book and how *painless* the transition was for the husband of a successful health author.

The key to understanding and accepting this sort of change is knowledge (to use the title of a book by Len J. Jones, *Ignorance is Not Bliss*), and if knowledge is the key, then desperation is the driving force.

Mary-Ann and I were desperate. Desperate for answers—answers backed by common sense and sound reasoning. Not the *do as I say, because I'm a doctor* sort of answer. We needed to understand what was going on here. Why were our bodies acting up? We knew that God in His wisdom did not make us with grommets in our ears and nor did He design us to rely on any of the thousands of superficial remedies or cures today.

Mary-Ann and I married in January 1977. I was working for Kentucky Fried Chicken at the time, and continued to work in hotels and restaurants for the next twenty years. I have always thought of myself as healthy, having played active sports all my life, but not as fit as I could be. But two maladies bothered me from when I was seventeen or eighteen years of age until I was thirty-three to thirty-four—severe indigestion and high blood pressure. These were explained as inherited from my parents; my dad continually suffered with indigestion, and my mom had a blood pressure problem. It irritated the hell out of me that I was penalized for having high blood pressure by the insurance companies when I was trying to take out coverage for my young family! Anyway, life goes on, and I had to live with the fact that every time I had my blood pressure taken, it was elevated for my age group and weight, and that there was nothing I, nor anyone else, could do about it—or so I thought.

Well, if you, too, believe that there are no solutions to these problems, let me tell you that you are wrong. These conditions are very easily explained and equally as easily rectified, and if you have the interest and resolve necessary to have gotten this far in this book, you'll be okay!

1984–85 were desperate years for us and our daughters; we were struggling with our health from all sides.

At this time we were eating all the health foods around; I was off coke (the soda version) and white bread, and into bran in a *big* way (I used to take tablespoons of the stuff and stir it into a glass of milk and force myself to drink this tasteless, coarse *gunge*), and despite all these radical precautions, we still managed to catch every flu, whether of the local or imported variety, and my youngest daughter had the proverbial *glazed donut* face constantly. Mary-Ann seemed to be doing her best to destroy our marriage with her mood swings, constant sneezing, rashes, and her interminable post-nasal drip.

I came across the book *Food Combining for Health* (Jean Joice and Doris Grant) and we put the principles of food-combining into practice and things started to change. And how they changed! My indigestion disappeared, never to return (except when I cheat), and Mary-Ann's many maladies cleared up within days. That was my first realization that there is more to this "diet thing" than just feeding our faces.

I'm not going to rewrite the book as all is basically said and done, but let me add that as a man, a husband, a father, and a businessman, you need your energy.

Energy is the secret to success.

Without it nothing gets done. No new ideas get implemented and no risks are taken. And without risk, no meaningful change or venture can be achieved, no goals can be reached, and, the bottom line is, nothing gets done! Think about it.

Think about your sex life for a second. Can you perform adequately for yourself and your wife if you don't have the energy to get off the couch? Can you get your business off the ground if you are being laid low with every bug that hits your neighborhood?

Jokes aside, sex is really important to most men, and the change to my diet resulted in radically improved performance and pleasure. But, if the transition to this lifestyle has done anything for me, it has given me energy. It has also helped me to understand this body that I will have to live in for the rest of my life.

It helped me to understand why I would on occasions get unexplainable anxiety attacks. When I had cleansed my system by eating correctly, I was able to isolate coffee as the culprit. I don't get these attacks anymore, and believe me, I work in a stressful environment. Today, I can have a cup of decaf coffee, I can have a beer or a glass of wine if I so choose (I do not drink alcohol at all now), but I never have more than two, simply because I am not prepared to spend a week (and I'm not joking) recovering from the after effects. In the past without realizing it I would just drink more coffee and sodas to keep me going or to recover from the effects of a few beers.

As far as the ubiquitous "business lunch" is concerned, it is very easy to say "I will stick to this or that" or "no dressing for me." These days colleagues are far less concerned when you have a "light" lunch than they were some years ago. Restaurants are far more accommodating about awkward requests, so don't let that put you off.

When I first switched over to this lifestyle, I would occasionally eat fish or chicken as part of my main meal. I have since lost the taste for animal flesh altogether and now prefer to meet my protein requirements by starting the average day with a quarter to half a cup of raw nuts blended with acid fruit in a "nut shake" (see recipe section or our Web site, www.mary-anns.com).

For lunch (that is, a working or business lunch) I'll have a salad (no dressing, no onion!) with a large baked potato with butter, and the vegetables of the day. (You may find it difficult at first to go without meat, in which case you could start with the salad and then go on to fish or steak of your choice—no fries or baked potato—and vegetables. Remember that all of this rigmarole becomes second-nature once you understand the basics of food-combining and have experienced the benefits of properly digested food.)

Mary-Ann handles "Making the Transition" to the Perfect Health lifestyle in the next chapter, but I feel that it is important to stress that the wake-up to lunch cycle should be strictly followed. I have found through bitter experience that a big breakfast or toast and coffee before noon will set me back for days. Business breakfasts are becoming increasingly popular these days. If you have to attend a working breakfast at any stage, start with fresh fruit, then sit back and listen or talk for an hour before you eat something else. Open that gap between meals for better digestion where you can.

Look, there has to be a certain amount of experimentation on your part, but the important thing is to fully grasp the principles. If you go off the rails once in a while, it is not a train wreck; you just get back on track as soon as you can.

Also (and most importantly) I find that exercising first thing in the morning does wonders. First, you don't particularly feel like eating much after a good workout so you can avoid the eating-too-much-too-early trap. Secondly, regular exercise is essential for vibrant health and tip-top energy levels. Today I walk between twenty and fifty miles a week and I try to spend time on my off-road motorcycle or in the garden, and even if I miss a day or two due to poor weather, I am able to resume my program where I left off without any ill effects.

Closing Tips

Most importantly, don't let your peers put you down! They won't ride the ambulance with you when you have your first heart attack!

And remember, guys, it is not just the lengths of our lives that is at stake here, it is the quality. Fewer ailments and aches and pains mean more productivity, and more productivity means more time for recreation and your family...and, if that ain't important to you, then make sure you are well insured so that your family can live comfortably without you and have money to pay the plumber and the handyman when you are gone.

CHAPTER SIXTEEN

Making the Transition

BY NOW you are probably overwhelmed. "Where do I start?" I can hear you say.

This chapter will, I'm sure, help you to make the transition as painlessly as possible. The key to changing your present, toxic, dietary lifestyle to one that is conducive to energy and health is not to try changing overnight. It is a rare individual who can do away with lifelong eating habits overnight and never look back. These few are to be commended. For the rest of us, a slow, gradual change is the answer.

Those of you who can make an immediate and total change might find that for the first week or two you will feel very tired. You may also find that your stomach is either upset or constipated, or that you have headaches. In fact, you may even develop strong flu-like symptoms. It is best not to take any medication for these symptoms, however, but rather to rest and get to bed as early as possible. These unpleasant reactions are merely due to cutting stimulants such as tea or coffee out of the diet or any other non-food toxic substance and it is the body's way of purging itself of residual toxins. In my experience, very few people have any of these symptoms for longer than seven days, although most only suffer for a day or two. This is one of the reasons so few people jump in with both feet and prefer rather to make gradual changes. If you do get any of these symptoms, you are not dying, only detoxifying! Take it slowly until you feel better.

Follow some hints for making the change without experiencing too much stress.

This Is Not a Diet, It Is a Lifestyle

Do not think of this way of eating as a diet. A *diet* is something you start and then stop. This is a new lifestyle that you are choosing. One cannot change a lifestyle overnight. It took you your entire lifetime to develop your existing habits. It takes time to change those habits, especially if you want permanent change.

Know That a Lifelong Lifestyle Cannot Be Changed Overnight

Old habits die hard is a most appropriate cliché at this point. The worst thing that you can do is to feel guilty about not being able to change your whole way of life overnight. Determine from the beginning that it is going to take some time, at least six months and maybe even a couple of years before you feel totally comfortable with your new way of life and altered eating patterns. A few years is a very short time compared to the many years it has taken you to result in poor health and weight gain. But take heart, you will start feeling the benefits immediately, or at least after two weeks. Some people only start responding positively to a change in diet after a two-week period of cleansing and detoxification. Do not get despondent if you suffer from the unpleasant symptoms of detoxification. This is probably the last time you'll ever feel like this again! Even if you go through detoxification more than once it is seldom as bad as the first time.

With Each Month That Passes, Strive to Improve Your Overall Diet

Make up your mind that with each month that passes, your diet will be a little better than it was the previous month. Even if that only means that instead of eating pizza every other night, you now eat it every third night. Small improvements lead to more complete health. You are the better for it, no matter how gradual the change.

This Is Not a "Give-Up" Diet, It Is an "Add-To" Diet

Do not think in terms of sacrificing—*I have to give up this and that—all the things I enjoy so much. I would rather eat the way I want to and die sick, but happy.* The emphasis should be on adding to your existing diet—adding more raw fruits and vegetables, rather than giving up the acid-forming "nice" foods you presently enjoy. As your body chemistry changes, your desires and cravings for foods will also change. Smokers often respond to this change by no longer feeling like a cigarette—to their amazement. Try introducing one step at a time and then when you are comfortable with that step introduce another.

Know That Wrong Cravings Will Eventually Be Fewer and Further Apart

As you gradually, but steadily, improve your diet, your body chemistry will begin to improve. The result will be that your desire for stimulation (toxic foods) will decrease just as gradually. Instead of craving pizzas three times a week, it will be just twice a week. Once you add more fruits and vegetables, natural foods, and essential fats to your diet for some time, your cravings for other foods will be less frequent.

Cravings for Good Foods Will Increase with Time

No matter how boring the very thought of a predominantly raw fruit and vegetable diet may seem, know that as the body chemistry changes toward a more alkaline, healthy chemistry, your desires and cravings for fresh and raw food will continually increase. These foods will become more palatable and you will wonder how you ever managed without them.

Eat as Well as You Can, for as Long as You Can

You may get really motivated to follow Perfect Health. You get started, you do well for three days, and then an overwhelming craving for a pizza hits you. If you can resist, great! If you can't, eat the pizza (just try and eat some raw vegetables before hand), and the next day get back on the diet for as many days as you can until a craving takes over again. I find that the three-day-craving rule is a great help. Try putting off what you are craving for three days—if you still feel like it on the third day, you deserve it! Take care that you do not over-indulge. It is not worth it—just make sure you eat some raw vegetables before the meal or fresh or preservative-free dried fruit before the candy or cookies.

Do Not Feel Guilty for Not Sticking to the Lifestyle 100 Percent

The worst thing you can do, literally worse than not eating the right foods, is to feel guilty when you break the lifestyle because of an old craving. Your body is punished when you eat badly so why punish yourself mentally, as well? Keep in mind that you cannot change a lifestyle and a body chemistry overnight. Apply this rule to exercise as well. If you don't make it today, don't feel guilty—go for a walk with your dog or do some sit-ups, and get out and work at it the following day. I find that having a mini-trampoline is a great help. After a couple of minutes of good bouncing, I feel that I have at least done some worthwhile exercise for the day.

A Reward System Is Often Beneficial

Some people have found that they can stick to the diet more diligently by making deals with themselves—*once a week (or month), I will have a splurge, I will eat anything I want, but for the rest of the time, I will follow the diet exactly.* Taking the family to a restaurant once a month and giving them the run of the menu, so to speak, is very effective. Over the years I have watched my family make healthier and healthier choices without any pressure on them to do so. We now have a rule where you can eat anything you like on your birthday and as our children have grown up those birthdays have become healthier. This works particularly well if you are changing the eating patterns of the whole family. But don't overdo it. Just remember that the healthier you become, the less you will need these splurges, and the worse you will feel afterward. Every indulgence will have its price.

Don't Be Too Stupid to Get Well

If you feel terrible after a splurge, or if you wake up with a *food hangover* the next morning, know that your body is now too healthy to tolerate certain foods. Continuing to splurge and getting sick afterward is an act of total stupidity, and good health will be slow in following. Listen to your body and make the changes it needs. I found the taste of refined sugar in my mouth was not worth the mood swings or depression the next day and that has always made it easier to make better choices.

Look Back Continually

What we tend to do when changing our eating patterns is to look forward to how far we still have to go. This can be very discouraging. Rather, take time, once a month, to look back at how far you have come. Take stock of how much your overall diet has improved since you first began eating healthier. You may, for example, have not eaten any fruit for days or weeks on end and now you are eating at least one or two portions a day! Looking back is far more encouraging and motivating and it will help you to stay on track.

Do Not Stock the Fridge and Pantry with "No-No's"

If junk foods are not readily available, they are not so easily eaten. If you have to make a special effort to run down to the grocery store in the middle of the night to get ice cream or chocolates, you may be deterred. This is a helpful suggestion for households that are attempting to change the children's diet; if the junk isn't in the house, they can't eat it. If they want it, they must provide their own transportation and money to get it. This is so important as they learn that they can take responsibility for what they eat.

Do Not Become a Martyr or a Fanatic

Nothing is more off-putting than a fanatic—one who says, "Look at me, I'm different and what's more, I'm better than you." Neither do people care for a martyr whose message is, "Poor me, I'm making the supreme sacrifice of diet to improve my health. Don't you feel sorry for me?" Both of these approaches reflect an attitude of pride and are counter-productive as people will be irritated both by you and your diet. In turn, this sort of negative feedback will discourage you and you may be tempted to give up the whole thing. Rather, don't be afraid to socialize and to eat a wrong thing or two now and then. Know instead that as time goes on and as this diet becomes more a part of you, your different lifestyle will not be offensive to others. It may become a point of interest and curiosity rather than one of irritation. You may find yourself, as many do, really helping others.

Never Give Advice if It Is Not Asked For

Ask me, I know! No matter how tempting it is to tell a parent he or she should not be giving his or her child diet soda (or any soda for that matter) in the child's bottle (or any other container) don't tell them.

I vividly remember sitting behind two mothers at my daughter's school just after I had realized that cow's milk was causing their tonsillitis and ear infections. They were bemoaning the fact that their children were continually on antibiotics and it was costing them so much money and time. I leaned forward to tell them to take dairy products out of their diet and I will never forget the way they looked back at me in absolute disdain and disgust. Yet what I was telling them would have solved the problem. I have realized throughout the years that until people are ready to make the change, it does not help how many success stories, facts, research, or arguments you offer them, they will not change. Rather focus on your own health and get on with your life. In time your glowing health will speak volumes and inspire those who are ready for change.

How to Convert an Unwilling Family to Healthy Eating

In the case of the mother (or person who prepares the meals) wanting to make the change of lifestyle, the best approach is not to warn the family that they are about to find strange, new meals on their plates. (The exception of course is if the family already has an excellent, above-average level of communication and if the children are very responsive to authority.) A subtle approach works far better. Without comment, over a period of months, ensure that the meals gradually become more nutritious. In addition to the regular meat serving, introduce lightly steamed vegetables and raw vegetable strips (crudités) with a dip. Ensure that fewer dairy products, fried foods, red meats, pre-prepared foods, and canned foods appear on the table. The most important step is to start by cutting out all brands of foods containing preservatives and other additives or artificial sweeteners. This is essential.

The next step is to serve a meal without meat or dairy products once or twice a week. Make no comment about the omission, just sit down and carry on as usual. If you do comment, you could find strong resistance. Just take it slowly. You will find that this gradual approach will ensure that even the most reluctant family members will become accustomed to the new, healthier habits in time.

In the case where Mom and Dad agree on the diet change, the transition is much smoother. Still, the less fanfare the better; just introduce more nutritious menus slowly, and set a good example by eating and enjoying without negative comment. Rather, make positive comments about how good the vegetables taste as they are being eaten, and how good they are for the body. If questions are raised as to why the menus are different, be honest and direct: "We've been reading (or the doctor told us, or John and Mary have been telling us) that junk foods make our bodies sick." I have found that by apologizing to the children for having fed them junk actually earned more respect. Follow with statements on how much better you have been feeling since eating properly, and comment on any change noticed in the children's health or behavior with the improved diet.

Don't neglect an opportunity to point out to the children when a slip away from healthful eating results in direct negative physical discomfort, both in you ("Boy, that ice cream sure gave me a headache") and in them ("Johnny, see how you are acting since you've eaten that cake"). Remember to remove all artificially preserved, sweetened, and colored foods, then introduce a bit of raw food at each meal.

At breakfast, start with a small fruit salad or plate followed by their "normal" breakfast. Eventually they will say that they are full from the fruit and will give the cereals or pancakes a miss. Cut a few slices or strips of tomato, avocado, cucumber, or carrot sticks and serve them with each meal as a slow introduction to raw food. I find that strips of raw vegetables served with mashed avocado or hummus before a meal are enjoyed by the whole family, and in particular by the children.

Don't Force Anyone to Eat Foods He or She Dislikes

Don't force children (or adults for that matter) to eat a particular vegetable because you think they need it. Be happy they are eating some vegetables even if it is only cucumber. Even if they will not eat any vegetables but do eat fruit, it is a start. I once met a mother who was in a state because she said her son would not eat any fruit or vegetables. I asked the son (who was nineteen) if there was any plant food he would eat and he said only cucumber and watermelon. I then encouraged him to eat some of each daily. Find one thing that they will eat; it is a starting place.

Hints on Socializing without Offending Your Health or Your Friends

You may find that once you and your family have made the adjustment to the Perfect Health lifestyle, you will all cope very well in the home. But what happens when a social situation arises?

HOW TO EAT AT A RESTAURANT

Restaurants can be a veritable minefield of potential problems, but there is no need to sabotage your health or to spoil your fun. We always start with a fresh salad, and ask the waiters to leave the dressing off as they seldom have any idea what it is made from themselves. We are not prepared to take a chance as many dressings are preserved with sulfur dioxide, which can cause hives and flu-like symptoms. If you like a tang to your salad, ask for plain oil and a fresh lemon and use this instead of the usual dressing. Try to order foods that are the least acidic and try to eat meals in good combination. Order salad and a baked potato, or salad and pasta, or salad and fish, or even just salad. Go for the neutral veggies or choose a pasta dish. If comments are made, say, "I'm just not that hungry, thank you." Don't be afraid to say, "It looks good, but I'm trying to change my lifestyle and it is making me feel so much better."

HOW TO BE A GOOD GUEST

Sharing a meal with friends is not reason to panic. At potluck dinners, go for the salads and vegetables and if you need to add a starch or a protein, who's going to notice? When sitting around a table, take the smallest portions and try to combine correctly. If you are planning to have the dessert, stick to carbohydrates during the main course—your stomach can handle this combination better than that of a protein followed by dessert. If you are in a position where you cannot avoid eating toxic foods or poor combinations, one helping will do. The body can, without too much cost, handle this occasionally if the digestive system is not overloaded. However, what we tend to do when the opportunity arises is eat far too much. It is actually harder on the body to overload in this manner than to eat incorrectly but moderately every day.

We found that eating a good salad before we go out takes the edge off our appetite, so that when we arrive at the venue we do not eat everything in sight. We also found feeding our children their favorite meal (usually spaghetti with homemade tomato sauce) before a party stops them from tucking into all the junk at parties. If you fill yourself beforehand with the good or better stuff, chances are your appetite will be pretty satisfied and you can eat small portions just to be polite. This also helps when you are only served dinner at nine or ten o'clock at night!

HOW TO ENTERTAIN HEALTHILY

When inviting others to your home, keep it simple. Fortunately there is a strong move away from rich complicated catering, not only at home but also in restaurants. It has in fact become quite fashionable to be health-conscious.

When planning your menu, it is best to cater for yourself first and then for your guests. In other words, let the focus of the meal be on alkaline-forming dishes such as salads and vegetables rather than having the table groaning with meat dishes. (Even the World Health Organization says that animal products should be regarded as the condiments to a meal.) If you must have a barbecue, go to town on the salads and try to serve only one kind of meat. A stir-fry barbecue is the ideal compromise. Prepare mounds of vegetables of your choice, including mushrooms, red peppers, bean sprouts, carrots, and celery, by cutting the vegetables into thin strips suitable for stir-frying. In addition, you could also prepare the meat or chicken beforehand by slicing it into thin strips as well. Then all you need for a successful barbecue is a large flat cooking surface, heated from below. A wok-shaped barbecue surface or even a flat griddle is ideal. Guests then proceed to cook their own meals by stir-frying whatever combination they like. This is a very sociable form of entertaining and it is an easy way to stick to good combinations. Vegetables done on or in the fire are delicious as well. Our favorite is potato done in foil. I wrap the potatoes in wax-wrap or grease-proof paper first (this prevents contamination of the food by aluminum) then in foil. Other vegetables we enjoy prepared in this way are corn on the cob, broccoli, fresh asparagus, butternut squash, and mushrooms. Add a bit of butter or cold-pressed olive oil and some seasoning of your choice and it's quite delicious. In fact you don't even need meat at a barbecue to enjoy the occasion.

Our favorite evenings are spent with friends around the table enjoying a properly combined meal. To give you some idea of how to go about this, here is a brief description of what I might serve for a casual supper:

When serving snacks or a starter, I go for crudités (fresh vegetables such as carrots and cucumber cut into strips) served with a dip. We prefer avocado dips and hummus although a ricotta cheese-based dip is also quite nice (make sure you have one that is dairy-free for people who are dairy intolerant) and an eggplant or mushroom pâté is even nicer. We might also serve some plain salted potato chips with the dips. (Potato chips are deep fried and therefore not ideal, but they pass as a cheat for special occasions.) Check that they contain no MSG (monosodium glutamate) or other additives. I also prefer the organic selection that is now available.

Our main course is more often than not a pasta and vegetable dish (a better combination than pasta and meat), always accompanied by a large, fresh salad. The vegetable sauces I find most popular are a home-made tomato sauce (Napolitano) and a creamy mushroom sauce made with fresh organic cream. I might also serve a loaf of freshly baked whole wheat bread with butter cut into cubes (the girls loved doing this for me). In fact, we always included our children in the preparation of all our meals, with Mark making the salad, the girls setting the table, cut-ting the butter, slicing the crudités, and making the dip, and with me as the director and maker of the main course. This is one of the reasons they grew up knowing how to entertain and how to prepare food prop-erly. If you have sons, involve them in the kitchen. You will be surprised at how they love it. We have had our grandsons in the kitchen from birth in their baby seats and now they love helping (imagine what great husbands they will make one day!). With the pasta dish I sometimes serve a bowl of grated Parmesan or pecorino cheese for sprinkling on top. Although this is not ideal from a food-combining point of view, it does add that little bit extra to the meal and it won't cause too much harm. Those who are dairy intolerant should skip the cheese.

Dessert

Dessert after any meal is not ideal as it usually has a high sugar content that, on top of the rest of your meal, will ferment in your stomach. If you serve dessert, a simple one free of preservatives and colorants is best. Dessert tends to ferment less when eaten after a starch, as opposed to a protein, meal. Serving dessert is not obligatory these days, but if you feel that you must, remember that the simpler the dessert, the bet-ter. I often place a bowl of fresh dates on the table instead of after-din-ner mints. We also do a dish of baked bananas with raisins, cinnamon, and honey, served with fresh organic cream. Grilled polenta slices with cinnamon, honey, and cream beat any waffle or pancake and are gluten-free. (See recipe section in Chapter Eighteen).

Casual Lunches

For a casual lunch we serve various breads such as rye, whole wheat, rice, or corn crackers and dips, and of course, plenty of salads. Whole wheat pita bread stuffed with salad is a firm favorite and for a delicious gluten-free meal we love grilled polenta slices served with grilled veg-etables and mashed avocados.

Formal Meals

A more formal dinner could consist of a vegetable starter such as steamed asparagus and hollandaise sauce, lemon butter, or our favorite, red pepper mayonnaise. Grilled black mushrooms, plain or stuffed with any mixture of vegetables, are another tasty starter. Avocado is a winner. Half an avocado scooped out and mashed or cubed with tomato, olives, celery, and feta cheese also goes down well. Alternatively, fresh stuffed tomatoes are a light, tasty starter. Just scoop out the flesh, dice it, and mix with fresh chopped basil, salt and pepper, avocado, or feta cheese (organic and optional) and olives, and return the mixture to the shell.

The main course would always have a fresh, crisp salad including any and every vegetable you like. Lightly steamed vegetables such as broccoli, cauliflower, and mushrooms are always interesting and tasty. Serve these with grilled sole or deep-water fish. Grill the fish on a baking sheet, dotted with butter, drizzle with freshly squeezed lemon or lime juice, and sprinkle with salt and pepper. Grill for approximately fifteen minutes. Or you could serve spinach-and-mushroom-stuffed savory buckwheat pancakes instead of the fish.

Entertaining at home the Natural Way should be easy and fun. Remember to keep it simple, spend time making the table attractive, and present the food with love and care.

How to Cater for a Children's Party

I find that many mothers battle with children's parties, but with a little lateral thinking, you will find that an ice cream cake, sodas, and brightly colored candy and cookies need not be the only options.

Popcorn is popular with any age group. Using a dry popper is best, but cold-pressed extra-virgin coconut oil can be used quite safely (and tastes spectacular) and butter is fine provided you resort to this method of preparation only on the odd occasion. (Remember that heated fats are not all that good for the body.) I always drizzle popcorn made in a popcorn machine with olive oil and then lightly sprinkle it with herbal salt. Plain, salted chips, although not ideal, can also be served. Go for the unflavored organic chips as one never knows exactly what is used in the flavoring and MSG is common. Unsalted, unroasted nuts are good savory alternatives, and bowls of cashews, almonds, pecans, or macadamias are great treats for any child.

On the sweet side, a good carrot cake is a winner, and for birthday parties it can be cut into any number of shapes and iced. (See recipe in the next chapter.) Carob cake is a good alternative to the usual chocolate cake and is, of course, much healthier. (See recipe in next chapter.) Dates, raisins, and preservative-free dried fruit are also popular. Of course, oat bars or cookies always go down well especially when dipped in melted carob. I have included a wheat-free recipe in the next chapter as well as one containing wheat flour. They are both delicious. Date and coconut balls are a lot of fun and tasty, too. (See recipe.) You can indulge occasionally and have real sweets if you must, but go for those containing no preservatives or artificial coloring. You will just have to live with the effect they have on your children.

A great way to start the party is to set out bowls of fruit salad or trays arranged with a variety of colorful fruits cut into squares. Include some toothpicks for the fun of it. Kids also love melon balls, especially if you do all three colors (pink, green, and orange).

Have the trays ready as the children arrive, and once they have eaten the fruit, let them play for a while before you bring out the other goodies. (This will allow the fruit to digest before they tuck into the rest of the food.)

Whole rye or whole wheat breads and biscuits, as well as pita bread, are more substantial snacks. Although hotdogs are out, homemade pizzas with or without cheese (see recipes), corn on the cob, and tacos (preservative- and additive-free) filled with a salad are filling and nourishing. Set out some whole wheat bread rolls with cubed butter, grated uncolored cheese, large grilled black mushrooms, mashed avocados, tomato slices, and lettuce, and let them make their own properly combined burgers using the mushroom as the patty. (Include the cheese for those who don't eat mushrooms.) You can also make a vegetable patty from mixed mashed vegetables combined with mashed potatoes and use these.

Instead of the usual fizzy sodas, serve juices that are free of preservatives or added sugar and add sparkling mineral water for the fizz. Ice cream can be served if you must, but look for a pure and organic brand or make your own. Ice cream is easy to make and is always popular. Take two cups fresh organic cream and one can of coconut cream (preservative-free) and blend together in your food processor with one cup of raw honey and a teaspoon of natural vanilla essence. Freeze the mixture for a couple of hours until set, remove, and blend again. Refreeze, remove, and blend. Freeze once again and serve—you will agree, it is delicious! Although this is an additive-free treat, it is very high in ani mal fat, which is not particularly good for the body, so make this only occasionally.

Parties don't have to be complicated. I have often prepared far too many dishes, realizing afterward that a more simple approach would have been better. So often we don't want to deviate from the norm and end up serving the usual hotdogs, hamburgers, and ice cream. Be daring, be different, be first! I have yet to see children not enjoying a healthy party. Keep thinking laterally and you'll come up with some great healthy ideas! (For more sugar-, wheat-, and egg-free dishes see the Perfect Health Digimag, which you can order from www.mary-anns.com. And look out for the Perfect Health recipe book.)

You will find it rather difficult to combine correctly at a children's party. Just do your best and get back on track the next day. So often we think that if we can't combine properly we might as well go the whole way and just serve total junk. Try to stick to the basic Perfect Health principles, and you will find that there will be no unpleasant repercussions.

Food-Grading Criteria

I have found that being able to grade food is very helpful when trying to decide which sorts of foods are healthier than others. In other words, by using the food-grading criteria, you will be able to see that a baked potato is far healthier than a roasted one and you will be able to make the best decisions for your health when faced with a choice. It is a simple and effective system that will be of great benefit to you when making the transition to the Perfect Health program.

FOOD-GRADING—THE ABC's OF FOODS

All foods can be graded into four simple categories (based on fresh, raw, and whole qualities):

- **A Foods**—these are fresh, raw, and whole (whole foods are those in their natural state). Seventy-five percent of the diet should be made up of these foods, which include all fresh fruit and vegetables. In other words, 75 percent of your food budget should be spent at the fruit and vegetable section of the supermarket

- **B Foods**—these have only two criteria. For example, a baked potato is fresh and whole, but not raw, as are all cooked vegetables
- **C Foods**—these are only fresh, only raw, or only whole. In other words, they have one criterion only. For example, unpolished rice is whole, but not fresh or raw
- **D Foods**—these have none of the above criteria. For example, potato chips or fries are neither whole, nor raw, nor fresh. Even within the D foods group there are healthier choices: whole wheat bread is better than white bread, and oat and coconut cookies are better than shop-bought, center-filled cookies

Buying, Storing, and Preparing Real Food

Once food-grading has become second-nature to you, and once you have made the best choices for your health, you must ensure that you do not destroy valuable nutrients inadvertently by the incorrect storage and preparation of your food. Here are some helpful tips to ensure that you derive the most benefit from your diet:

- Buy produce as close to ripe as possible. It is cheaper and you know that it will ripen properly
- Do not buy foods that will not rot as these contain a preservative of some kind. Long shelf life foods should also be avoided as they are usually not as nutritious as fresh foods
- Do not buy foods that have been irradiated. Irradiation has been shown to cause carcinogenic and mutagenic changes in foodstuffs, as well as destroy vital nutrients—avoid them
- Do not buy foods that contain any additives, including colorants and artificial flavors
- Buy foods as close to their natural state as possible. For example, don't buy any ready-peeled vegetables or pre-prepared salads. These are often treated with a sulfur-based preservative and once cut, nutrients are lost rapidly
- Wash your fruits and vegetables carefully with an environment-friendly soap to remove any residual fertilizers or insecticides
- Store vegetables that don't have skins (such as lettuce and cabbage) in air-tight containers or plastic bags
- Steaming is the best way to cook—this method destroys the least amount of nutrients

- Waterless cooking is second-best
- Stir-frying is a good method if water, instead of oil, is used. This is done very easily and effectively; stir fast and control the temperature
- Roasting and baking are also good methods of preparation as there is no water involved to carry away nutrients. Bear in mind, though, that extreme temperature can destroy some nutrients. So slower roasting and baking for a longer period of time is better
- Avoid boiling as it robs food of nutrients
- Avoid aluminum foil and pots, and non-stick cookware that is scratched or damaged as these substances oxidize easily if damaged, so get rid of any pots or pans that have deep scratches. They can contaminate the food during the cooking process, and the contaminants can get into the bloodstream
- Avoid all fried foods. The body cannot cope with heated fats
- Try not to use a microwave oven—this method of cooking destroys as many nutrients as pressure cooking or vigorous boiling. And there is always the danger of leakage from the microwave. Stand at least six feet away from a microwave if you do use it
- Use as few condiments as possible

Making the transition from your old habits to the Perfect Health lifestyle is not as difficult or as complicated as you may have feared. Take things slowly and don't become discouraged if you are not able to progress as quickly as you would like. Try to stick to the Perfect Health principles whenever you can—turning to the hints and suggestions outlined in this chapter will encourage you and will help you stay on track.

Remember that you only have to make better choices one meal at a time.

As far as your new eating patterns are concerned, keep it simple; keep it healthy; and have fun making better choices one meal at a time.

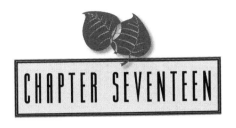

CHAPTER SEVENTEEN

Success Stories
Changing to the Perfect Health Lifestyle

"Success is not measured by what a man accomplishes, but by the opposition he has encountered and the courage with which he has maintained the struggle against overwhelming odds."

—CHARLES LINDBERGH

IN THIS CHAPTER, I have included the most dramatic transformations that various people have experienced when changing their lifestyles to a more natural and healthy one. No two people are the same; we inherit different metabolisms and our internal organs function at different rates. But each person whom I have dealt with, who has managed to stick to the Perfect Health program at least 80 percent of the time, has experienced a dramatic improvement in health and energy—although some progressed faster than others.

It is not likely to be smooth sailing when you make the changes; you may be criticized by those you know and love. You need to build a circle of friends that has the same values and goals as you. You are also likely to experience some unpleasant detoxification symptoms and reading these stories will inspire you to keep going.

Melanie

Melanie had been a vegetarian for many years but her level of health was quite poor. She came to me slightly overweight and suffering from frequent migraines that struck two to three times a week. She had been on antibiotics for her skin, she had been taking laxatives for fifteen years, as well as antacids almost daily for indigestion, the odd tranquilizer for tension, and the occasional paracetamol painkiller for, as she put it, twitches. She had also resorted to using cortisone cream daily for a troublesome skin rash. After a two-week cleansing program of just raw fruit, vegetables, and nuts (during which she suffered from detoxification symptoms such as nausea, migraines, and general discomfort for two to three days), Melanie felt like a new person. Her stomach was working regularly and comfortably without the aid of a laxative for the first time in fifteen years, she came within her goal weight, her energy levels had improved, she found that she could cope with stress far better than before, and her skin had improved. The indigestion, previously her constant companion, had also disappeared. Of course, everything did not improve overnight, or even in the first two weeks. But during the last nine months, she has stuck to the maintenance program (a high-raw diet with properly combined foods, and no additives) 80 percent of the time, and Melanie's skin continues to improve as do her general health and well-being.

Dennis

Dennis was in his sixty-eighth year when he came to see me. As his wife Hanna put it, "Dennis has been tired since we got married." Dennis had suffered a heart attack six years before, was slightly anemic, overweight, and suffered daily from reflux problems that were accompanied by vomiting. After six weeks on the maintenance program combined with regular exercising on a rebounder (mini-trampoline), Dennis had his blood tested and found that he was no longer anemic. His energy levels had improved drastically, and to quote Dennis, "I have more energy than I've ever had." The hernia attacks had also become milder and further apart. Now, nearly a year later, Dennis has not had a hernia attack for many months, even though he "cheats" occasionally. I would like to mention here that Dennis has had the support of his wife Hanna, who joined him in the change to a natural, healthy lifestyle. I'm sure that without her, he would have struggled. Hanna, by the way, has also experienced an improvement in her health and well-being.

Barry

Barry, thirty-seven years old, came to me because his cholesterol was too high (9.2 m/mol). He was also slightly overweight, had low energy, and suffered from indigestion. Within a month Barry had lost weight, his cholesterol was down dramatically, his energy had shot up, his general health had improved considerably, and his indigestion disappeared.

Terence

Terence, three years old, was brought by his mother to see me. Terence had recurring pneumonia. Antibiotics could not clear this up and his mother was told that he would have to be hospitalized as this condition had persisted for six months. His mother was convinced that he would not leave the hospital alive. I put Terence on a cleansing diet for two weeks. For the first two days, all he consumed were water and freshly extracted fruit juice—he wasn't hungry and refused all food. He slept for three hours in the morning and another two to three hours during the afternoon. By the third day he was eating a little fruit and sleeping less. Each day his appetite increased and eventually he was sleeping for only two hours during the afternoon. Two weeks later he was running about, rosy-cheeked and full of energy. On the Perfect Health program he remained off all meat and dairy products (other than butter). He ate no foods containing artificial additives and he was feeling so well that he did not need to visit the doctor. On the odd occasion when he ate incorrectly (at a birthday party for example), his face became a bit drawn and his nose would run for two to three days. Terence has now grown into a healthy twenty-one-year-old studying sports science at college and has remained healthy and fit.

Joyce

Joyce, sixty years old, arrived feeling that life was passing her by. She had no energy and sweated profusely for no apparent reason. If you had met Joyce, you would've realize how embarrassing this was for her— she was always beautifully dressed and immaculately groomed. Joyce wanted to be off her medication as well as lose some weight (to be down one dress size, as she put it). Since being on the Perfect Health program for the last one and a half years, she has lost weight and her energy has improved drastically. She no longer gets headaches or takes laxatives, diuretics, or appetite suppressants. To put it in Joyce's own words, "Life is so uncomplicated now."

Merle

Merle came to me in quite a state. She suffered from premenstrual tension accompanied by severe migraines that would force her to spend two days in bed each month. Part of her recurring problem was that she retained up to 6–7 pounds of water each month. Her doctor had put her on Evening Primrose oil, which caused diarrhea, a multivitamin, and a vitamin B6 supplement, but her breasts became enlarged and uncomfortable from these. She also suffered from severe pains in one of her kidneys, she felt full and bloated all the time, she had pains in her joints, and she had already had polyps on her gallbladder removed. Merle also craved sweets so badly that she would get up to raid the kitchen at midnight to try and satisfy her sweet tooth. Although she had been placed on a so-called "balanced" diet by a dietitian, and exercised almost daily, her problems persisted and her general health remained poor. After placing her on a correctly combined high fruit and vegetable diet, Merle's many problems have cleared up and she has remained in good health for well over a year.

Angelique

Angelique, who after years of being continually sick with bronchitis, sinusitis, and various bladder infections, decided she was literally sick and tired of taking pills. She showed me copies of three successive monthly medical bills submitted to her medical insurance—they were more than her monthly grocery bill. This was just a sample of her medical history that reflected deteriorating health throughout many years. Within a month of changing to the Perfect Health lifestyle, she felt like a different person and she has not had a medical bill since; she has found that she no longer enjoys smoking and after forty years has stopped! I am sure that her medical insurance is thrilled.

There are many others who have changed to the Perfect Health program who prefer to remain anonymous. I think of the fifty-three-year-old man who could not sleep uninterruptedly through the night without his stomach giving him tremendous problems with cramps and wind. He claimed that he went through a packet of antacids in less than a week. He now sleeps through the night and hasn't touched an antacid tablet since changing his eating habits.

Then there is the twenty-three-year-old man who said that he woke up feeling tired and then continued throughout the day in this exhausted state. He could sleep for twelve hours and yet still be tired when he awoke. By cutting out the so-called energy-giving drink that he consumed daily and by increasing the fresh fruit and vegetable content of his diet, he now has boundless energy and his stomach works regularly.

Many of the people I have counseled do not have disgusting eating habits, and in fact, most are quite health-conscious. If anything, their eating and exercise programs are just directionless and they have been confused by the snippets of various health philosophies they have tried to incorporate into their lifestyles. They have all found the Perfect Health program and its principles extremely easy to follow and very rewarding.

Below are some of the letters I have received via e-mail throughout the last fifteen years. I could truly go on and on, citing many more case studies, in fact I could fill a few books, but the message I'm trying to get across, indeed the purpose of writing this book, is that you can take responsibility for your own health and well-being—and that includes solving any weight problems. It is not difficult at all. Start slowly, make a change, however small, and commit yourself to it. The more you do, the easier it will become and the better you and your family will look and feel. Start now! Remember, your body will sort itself out if you let it.

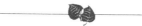

Dear Mary-Ann,

I want to thank you for the wisdom I gained by reading your books and the privilege I had in attending three of your lectures. From there I had to take it further on my own with the help of my heavenly Father.

First, my job was to read your books, which my youngest daughter gave me. Both of us have many allergies. I was diagnosed with chronic urticaria in 1997. My specialist prescribed medication for the rest of my life. My problem got worse as the years went by; I suffered from headaches and terrible itching. Sometimes I scratched until the skin was damaged and it then took a long time to heal. Not to mention the sneezing, blocked nose, itchy eyes, swollen ankles, and irregular heartbeat that missed five beats in a minute. I also suffered from constipation. I am a qualified nurse and a single mom, have raised three daughters, and was seventy years old last September. At the end of November we attended your lecture and bought The Natural Way. I was ready to reduce my medication, sleeping tablets, painkillers for arthritis, and blood sugar tablets. Believe me, it was not easy, but it can be done. My help was plenty of prayer and a change in diet by observing your five steps.

My health improved and as a bonus I have lost 7 pounds in three months.

Kind Regards,
Margaret

Dear Mary-Ann, Mark, and Family,

Two years ago I decided to go on Perfect Health. My cancer marker disappeared, I no longer suffer from migraine headaches, skin allergies (itchy dry skin), or whiteheads.

I wake up full of energy, having slept well—no sleeping pills, no medication! No visits to the doctor, although I do have a yearly gynecological check-up. Plenty of fresh, raw vegetables has proven to be a useful addition to my husband Jim's diet, which appears to have regulated his blood pressure, electrolytes, and heart function and improved his general health. Olive oil and flaxseed oil are compulsory in our daily consumption. Thank you for all the useful information.

I forgot to mention that three years ago I had recurring tonsillitis, and at the age of sixty-seven it is very dangerous to consider a tonsillectomy. Hence my search for an alternative, with good results! I've been through the winter every year since, without a cold or any sign of a sore throat!
Thank You Again,
Bev

Dear Mary-Ann,
I started your way of eating just over three months ago and cannot get over how wonderful it is. I heard you speak some years back but did nothing about it even though I had very high cholesterol. It would not come down with medication and the doctor told me it was hereditary and said I would need medication for life. I was also overweight and have never liked the idea of taking drugs. I started following your principles recently and have lost more than 20 pounds and my cholesterol is lower than ever before. I made the serious mistake of previously excluding all the good fats, thinking they would make me fat; well, they have not, as you can see, and they brought down my cholesterol just as you said. I also used to eat sugar to give me energy for exercising without realizing that it caused my mood swings and depression. I am forty-eight years old, am looking forward to a healthy menopause, and everyone is telling me how wonderful I look. Thank you so much. My only regret is that I did not make the changes earlier.
Lyn

Dear Mary-Ann,
I am fourteen years of age and am extremely thankful for what you and your book have done for me.

Early last year I was really hurting because I was continually being teased about my weight. I loved to eat donuts, cheese, cookies, junk food, coffee, tea, milk, sugar...sugar...sugar—in fact, anything and everything that was sweet.

My mom thinks that your way of eating is the healthy way, so she has your books on our bookshelf at home. I began to read The Natural Way and felt that this was something I could do.

I began to eat fruit and vegetables daily, drank lots of water, and ran for fifteen minutes every morning. It was difficult to do this at first but I guess I really needed to see a change in my situation. I weighed 130 pounds and since I have been eating fruit and vegetables, I weigh 100 pounds—the ideal weight for my age and height. I lost all of the weight in the first three months of following Perfect Health.

I feel great and never struggle to fit into clothes. I just want to thank you. I do home schooling and have decided that I want to help other children like me. I would like to study your course to become a Perfect Health consultant.
Thanks and Regards,
Hailey

(Hailey is the youngest student to have completed our Perfect Health Course.)

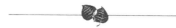

Hi Mary-Ann,
First of all, I want to tell you that to date I have lost more than 50 pounds, have lots of energy, and look fantastic. I am getting compliments wherever I go!
Thank You,
Bubbles

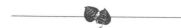

Hi Mary-Ann,
Just a short note to say it has been five weeks since we started living and eating the Natural Way (weekends have been the toughest time but are getting easier). We (my hubby, my two daughters, ages three years and eight months respectively, and myself) all have ten times more energy. My toddler has had very few temper tantrums. I lost 10 pounds in the first two weeks and have lost more since then, and

have lost two dress sizes! My confusion is gone, my concentration is
strong, and I feel amazing!
Thank you for saving our lives!
Maria, Michael, Gabrielle, and Isabella

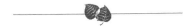

This is my story:
I have three children: Veronica is four, Michaela is two, and Declan is
four months old. Veronica has been our "doctor baby" from the begin-
ning—it started when she was five weeks old and was diagnosed as
lactose intolerant and I was told to stop breast-feeding her until her
stools became normal. Being a first-time mom and very ignorant, I
listened! Since then, she had a runny nose, tonsillitis, ear infections,
and a constant cough relating to a post-nasal drip. I was told that
she had baby asthma and with consistent antibiotics, nasal drops,
and an inhaler, she would eventually outgrow it. Michaela also had
her first ear infection and they were both fitted with grommets. Dur-
ing my quest to find the ultimate solution and not accept any more
medication, I came across The Natural Way and our lives changed.
On the first of April 2003, I took my two girls off dairy (milk, yogurt,
and cheese) and preservatives and gradually introduced the rest of
Perfect Health. Veronica's little body went through a bit of detox in the
first few months, but we persevered and have not looked back—it is
almost a year without an antibiotic in our house!

My children are vibrant, healthy, and have limitless energy! De-
clan is completely breast-fed and I will continue to breast-feed for
as long as I can. I am so passionate about this way of life that I will
be doing the nutrition course in the near future and will spread the
word to anyone who will listen—it just makes so much sense!
Thanks for making the books available to us all!
Regards,
Janine

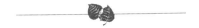

Hi there Mary-Ann,
I am writing this letter primarily to say thank you for writing your
books. If you hadn't, we may never have discovered the benefits of

the lifestyle you call Perfect Health. If I may share with you our story:

In January of this year, my wife Shirley was admitted to the hospital with what appeared to be a bad case of gastroenteritis. By about the sixth day in the hospital, after many tests and trauma, the doctors suspected ulcerative colitis (UC) and confirmed this with a colonoscopy. The relief of finally knowing what was wrong soon gave way to further stress and confusion about what this implied and how we were to deal with it. It was only through God's love and grace that we were able to cope with this stressful time. Shirley finally returned home after eight days in the hospital.

At that time, a friend loaned us your book, thinking that Shirley would benefit. Shirley read The Natural Way *during those two weeks at home, and when I think back I cannot believe how easy it was for us to make the change—it just seemed to happen. My initial and primary reason for changing to Perfect Health was to support Shirley and I was unprepared for how it would change my life, as well. I have never had any weight problems and have been blessed with reasonably good health for most of my life, but I have always suffered from mild asthma attacks, mostly exercise-induced, as well as hay fever, sinuses, and mucus-related problems such as bad post-nasal drip, etc. I will never forget the feeling of waking up in the morning—after about four days on Perfect Health—full of energy and feeling as sharp as a whistle. I felt better than I had felt in years! We have now been following this lifestyle (probably more than 80 percent of the time) for about six weeks. Shirley's ulcerative colitis seems to have gone into total remission. Shirley, who was initially nearly 20 pounds over her ideal weight, lost it all. As for myself, I have experienced a significant decrease in mucus-related problems, including post-nasal drip, and even lost about 5 pounds. Steele*

Hi Mary-Ann,

For my entire teenage and adult life I have never had a normal menstrual cycle. According to the textbooks normal means menstruating every twenty-eight to thirty-five days. My menstrual cycle was always forty-six-plus days. I started menstruating when I was fourteen and over the years my cycle remained inconsistent and premenstrual

syndrome got worse with age. I thought that suffering from Premenstrual Syndrome, blood sugar problems, and inconsistent menstrual cycles was something that I just had to endure. Seven years ago I changed to Perfect Health and became a vegetarian—I still ate wheat and dairy. I was also diagnosed with polycystic ovarian syndrome. Six months ago my premenstrual tension was getting so bad that I thought I would need anti-depressants. After speaking to Mary-Ann she advised me to go off wheat and dairy, which I did. Within the first month of cutting out wheat and dairy, my menstrual cycle was shortened to thirty-two days. I must admit, I was rather skeptical, initially, as to whether this would work, so I was really in a state of shock when my menstrual cycle shortened. Even though I had read your books I thought that it would not work for me. I had nothing to lose, so I gave it a try. I have remained off wheat and dairy because I feel so good. My PMS symptoms have vanished, I sleep less than I used to, and I do not have any blood sugar level drops/rises. What is also interesting is that I do not have that sweet/salty craving that used to plague me every month about ten days before a period. Water retention is a thing of the past, as is breast tenderness. What motivates me to stay off the wheat and dairy is that I do not want to experience the terrible symptoms I had before and I am stunned that for the first time in my life I am having a period every thirty-two days. For me, flaxseed oil is something I cannot live without. Even when I get ovarian pain, I use flaxseed oil as a means of pain relief. Flaxseed oil is an anti-inflammatory (as you explained to me) and within half an hour my ovarian pain is gone. I usually experience this ovarian pain during ovulation or just before a period. The other supplement that I could not live without is Barley Life. It has taken a bit of effort to change my diet but it has been so worthwhile. Thanks to you, my hormonal system is working a lot better, which has had an amazing effect on my body, mind, and spirit!
Jacqui

(Jacqui went on to have a healthy pregnancy and is raising her child on Perfect Health.)

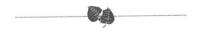

Hi Mary-Ann and Family,
I want to say thank you for all your wonderful research, advice, and mentoring.

My husband and I have been learning about and working toward health for the past three years now—and you have been such an inspiration to us. I followed your principles and advice for preparing for pregnancy. I had a wonderful pregnancy—loved it all—and such a special home birth with no problems at all and breast-feeding has been easy.

I used to have really bad periods and I know that all steps of my pregnancy would have been awful if not for your teachings. So many of our friends and family members have since also been blessed and inspired by the information in your books and tapes!

Best of all, our little Victoria Grace is so happy and healthy and such a joy to us! God is so good!

Thank you so much and God bless in all you are doing.
Love and Blessings,
Caryn, Morgan, and Vicki

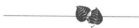

My name is Saiurie Naidoo; I'm nineteen years of age. My family and I (my mom, dad, and myself) have been following your program for about a year now and absolutely love it!

My mom found out about you last year and is totally engrossed and fascinated by your discovery of Perfect Health. She has read almost all your books and has learned a tremendous amount of valuable information! She has specifically asked me to express her gratitude to you as we are reaping the rewards of this diet and noticing the difference in our lives every day.

Thank you again for making such a difference.
All the best to you and your family.

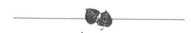

Hi Mary-Ann,
I am in New Zealand and my experience is as follows:

I have suffered with severe sinus pains in the cheeks, behind the eyes, toothaches, neck pains, back pains, extreme exhaustion, irritated eyes, etc. I went to every doctor imaginable in New Zealand and not one of them could pinpoint the cause. This went on for two and a half years at great expense, as my medical insurance would not cover me as it was a pre-condition according to them as I had previous sinus surgery.

- *GP's—pumped me full of antibiotics, nasal sprays, antihistamines*
- *Naturopath—handfuls of herbal medications, which did nothing*
- *Homeopath—same as above*
- *Dentist—could not find anything wrong*
- *Chiropractor—kept adjusting and adjusting and made no difference*
- *Acupuncture—worked for a while and then went back to being unbearable*
- *Allergy Specialist—tested for allergies extensively; all tests came back negative for airborne, food, and other. Also tested for a few specific ones such as pine, moss, and mold, as I seemed to have the strongest reaction around these, with no luck*
- *Pain Clinic—here they took me off all medications and tried to improve my posture, breathing, sleeping, diet, exercise. This helped for a period of three months, then went back to normal again*

The funny thing, in all of this, was no one suggested I go off wheat and dairy. I went off wheat and dairy for about three months after reading about allergies on the Internet and from speaking to various people. I did a detox diet for three months. The effects only lasted for a month or two and then I was back to square one.

I read your book at the beginning of October this year and it has changed my life.

I have not been on any medication since then, have not been to any doctors since then, have not had dairy, only a little bit of whole wheat bread now and again. I have boundless energy, go to the gym regularly, and work much better, as I am not so tired. And the real cherry on top is that I am no longer constantly dieting to control my weight. I have lost 15 pounds since October, have kept it off, and I know the rest will follow in good time.

Thanks so much for all your advice. It is so simple and logical. Keep up the good work!

Regards,

Erika

Dear Mary-Ann,

I was introduced to this lifestyle—Perfect Health—by my colleague, John, a dentist in the town of Hastings, East Sussex, England. John joined the practice in June 2001. Right from the beginning he shared enthusiastically the principles of the Perfect Health lifestyle with me and gave me a copy of your book to read. From the first day we met John, both Mr. Mann (another colleague) and I admired him for his high level of energy. John and I are the same age, but he was (and still is) so full of energy, that it seemed to me he was always running instead of walking. I will always be grateful to John for sharing this lifestyle with me and thankful to God for sending him to work with me.

I read the book while on holiday and I could not put it down. I often referred to it again and again (still do). I can now testify that I know where all of John's energy comes from. Since I have been following the principles of the book, I've experienced my energy levels rise. I used to take a nap every lunch break but now I have extended my lunch break to two hours and I am visiting the gym instead. I can recommend this book to every person who wants to improve his or her quality of life. My life has improved dramatically.

Since following the Perfect Health lifestyle and taking Barley Life and flaxseed oil (Aimega) daily, I haven't had any sickness or illness and if I do get flu-like symptoms (rarely), they don't last longer than a day or two. I was suffering badly from heartburn and indigestion—I haven't had any symptoms for more than a year now and I haven't had any medication whatsoever, I lost more than 40 pounds and am down three sizes to the size I used to wear ten years ago. I feel good about myself and I know I am absolutely doing the right thing. I have been taking Barley Life for more than three months and I can now feel that I am giving my body all the vitamins, minerals, and enzymes it needs to function optimally. Both my body and mind feel wonderful.

Thank you, Mary-Ann, for your books and all your support. I will never change this lifestyle for anything else and it is a privilege for me to honor God by looking after my body, His temple, and sending out this message to other people.

Jan

My story is as follows:

At the beginning of the year I was twenty-six, weighed nearly 300 pounds, and was in bad shape. I was taking a drug called Tofranil for a spastic bladder and using painkillers for headaches that would come and go. I also suffered from a number of smaller ailments such as sinus trouble and recurring flu. My diet was very bad, living on mostly take-out and junk food such as chips, sodas, and chocolates. I also used lots of milk and dairy products and was eating meat just about every night. These meals were badly combined as I found out after reading about it in The Natural Way, *which was the answer as to why I suffered from heartburn and indigestion all the time.*

Since putting the principles in The Natural Way *into practice I have lost 50 pounds, my sinuses have cleared up, I have a more regular heartbeat, I haven't had the flu for four months, I feel stronger and more energetic, sleep better, and have an overall feeling of better health. I also suffered from IBS (Irritable Bowel Syndrome) and using mostly Perfect Health principles, along with some additional guidelines, have managed to restore my digestive system to its original healthy state. In short, Perfect Health has saved my life because I don't think my body would have been able to endure the abuse it was receiving for much longer. It made me aware that your diet is crucial for a higher quality of life. The whole focus of Perfect Health is awareness. Be aware of what you are doing to your body. Living badly means you feel terrible and your business, social, and personal life are affected. Financially, I spent thousands to help my physical condition, which after following Perfect Health (some simple guidelines), I have managed to do better than any medication has helped me. In fact, I believe that the medication I was taking only aggravated the whole situation.*

God Bless,

Justin

(Justin has gone on to lose even more weight—another 60 pounds—and is at his ideal weight. He has also studied our Perfect Health Course and Consulting Course and is helping hundreds of people via the Internet on www.mary-anns.com.)

Hi All,

Just a quick note to first thank you and, second, encourage you to keep up the excellent work that God called you for. My name is Mari Venter; I turned thirty-two last month and I can honestly say that I feel a million times better than when I turned twenty-one. So far I've lost 60 pounds and the remaining 10 are on their way out, but more importantly, I feel like a new person.

I spent a couple of years jumping between calorie-controlled and high-protein diets such as Weight Watchers and Atkins—also diet milk shakes and pills, and, of course, BioSlim! None of these permanently budged the needle on my scale, so I decided to re-read The Natural Way given to me by my brother in 1999. I slowly started including the five steps while still eating whatever my body craved and subsequently ended up daily taking a handful of supplements (as I've learned now that I only supplemented the sewer system), which consisted of iron, zinc, chromium, vitamin B-complex, Centrum, echinacea, and additional vitamin C with L-lysine because I constantly had a mouthful of fever blisters. On top of all this my doctor prescribed 5mg Zopax twice daily to reduce my nervousness (stress).

After many mornings spent trying to swallow all these tablets and having the most awful aftertaste, I gave up; first, because since starting to take these supplements my "traveling pharmacy" grew daily to cope with the permanent headaches, constipation, nausea, and lethargy and second, my medical aid was pushed over the "threshold" with all these expenses. I knew I could not possibly continue living this way and since I was labeled as manic depressive a couple of years ago, I knew that the Zopax was going to be replaced or supplemented by either Aropax or Cipramil or one of the new wonder drugs if my despondency and gloominess continued.

When I started, my detox was severe for four or five days, but I began on a Wednesday so thankfully the worst occurred over a weekend and I could sleep it off. I got into the swing of things and decided that I wanted to try the additional products that you support so I got the Herbal Fiber Blend and Barley Life as well as Aimega blend of oil. The last two weeks of August I went completely raw and added five days of freshly extracted juice in between. I lost 10 pounds but more importantly I felt better than I have on any of my previous birthdays (including childhood because I grew up loving sweets).

Sadly I have to admit that last Tuesday I received a block of fudge of which I had a one-inch-square piece—thinking that I wasn't being too bad. Wrong. On Wednesday morning I woke up with a migraine from hell, my head spun, and my eyes burned so much that I pulled out half my eyelashes in an attempt to stop the itching. I had water the whole day—mostly because anything else I tried came out immediately and by Thursday I felt almost human again.

I definitely decided that nothing tastes good enough to justify feeling like that ever again!

My progress has been noted by people I work with and on Monday our director—a generous man named Chris Leal—agreed to sign me up to study your nutritional course. He took one of my copies of your book and the food-combining chart home and every day he says he just wants to read a bit more before bringing it back because he's had a digestion disorder since I started working here five years ago. I've mailed five copies of The Natural Way *to some of my colleagues all over the country, as well as products, DVDs, and all printed matter I can find to some of our in-house staff who all have the normal spastic colon, heartburn, allergies, all-year flu, etc., which everyone has come to accept as part of the modern lifestyle.*

I am looking forward to receiving my study material—and once again I'd like to thank you for being faithful to God's call in your lives.

May God bless you and your whole family every day.
Regards,
Mari Venter

Hi Mary-Ann,
At age twelve, I was brought to the Natural Way by my mother who had come across a Natural Way article in a Christian magazine.

Following a holiday in the Far East, I had an undiagnosable condition that had persisted for six months. I had clocked up thousands of dollars worth of medical bills and blood tests and consulted a number of top physicians and doctors. All to no avail—just utter confusion and desperation. With each blood test and new physician, came a new diagnosis—presence of Epstein Barr virus and CMV virus, tagged as recurring glandular fever; viral encephalitis;

Gilbert's liver syndrome; chronic fatigue syndrome; recurring Myal-gic encephalitis; and the list goes on.

Deep concern set in among my family as the weeks went rolling on, with no improvement in my health whatsoever. Chronic exhaus-tion, deep muscle aches and swellings, no toleration of anything besides work and bed. At the point where physicians were at a loss for prescribing how to manage the condition and resolving to book me off work for a couple of months, Mom purchased a copy of The Natural Way. Believing we had been led to the book through prayer, both Mom and I at once set about implementing the lifestyle...fer-vently! The incredible healing powers of raw (living) foods and Perfect Health food-combining were dumbfounding to all—me, my family, and the physicians/doctors I had been consulting. We found my body had begun healing itself literally within seventy-two hours of starting to implement Perfect Health. Within a fortnight the res-toration was clearly visible. After a month or two, nothing but up—all and only attributable to the miracle of Perfect Health!

Mom and I remain staunch subscribers of Perfect Health. For me, it is not only now the lifestyle of choice after its testimony in my life, but also the lifestyle of necessity. I find a momentary lapse to a looser diet resuscitates all the wretched symptoms. Thank you Mary-Ann, your book and wisdom were Godsends. I consider it such a privilege to have the knowledge of the Perfect Health lifestyle at my age and stage.

Jane

My story:

During July 2000 my husband and I were on holiday in the Berg. I was having constant diarrhea, so I tried to cut down on dairy products, which helped a little. When we got home I went to see the doctor. After numerous tests, which proved I did not have a bacterial infection, parasitic infection (tests in South Africa are quite useless in this regard by the way), or a milk allergy, I was diagnosed with Irritable Bowel Syndrome.

My symptoms matched the disease perfectly. I was put on a chronic prescription, costing hundreds of dollars a month. This helped, but did not take my symptoms away completely. I was to the point of suffering from chronic fatigue to the extent that I was unplugging my alarm clock in my sleep. I was also constantly sick, had terrible flatulence, was constantly bloated, and had permanent stomach pains. No matter how hard I worked out at the gym I just could not go beyond a certain performance level. Not only that, but I had resigned myself to the fact that at age twenty-two my metabolism was obviously slowing down and that middle-age spread had begun, because I could not lose weight no matter what.

I was also in a state of depression, often thinking that I was a little bit crazy. My concentration was very poor and my memory was terrible. I also had monthly recurring candida infections, which would be treated with antibiotics—much to my disgust. Things only got worse as over a period of a year I began to develop chest pains along my breastbone. I am a type-A personality—perfectionist tendencies, etc.—so I thought it was stress-related. I did every anti-stress thing you could imagine: taking herbal tranquilizers, showering with anti-stress shower gel, you name it, but nothing helped.

Eventually back to the doctor I went, this time to be sent for a gastrocope at the local hospital after which they diagnosed a burnt esophagus caused by acid reflux—again linked to stress, they said, and I just felt guilty that I was causing my own illness. After being put on another prescription for chronic medication (a lot more money) I decided to try to find other ways to combat this problem—I tried cutting out all acid-forming foods and followed every article written on indigestion. I eventually stopped the medication and went on herbal digestive enzymes to help me with the digestion of my food. This helped to an extent, about the same as the expensive medication, but I was still tired, overweight, sick, and not very happy about having to take a tablet before every meal I ate.

Eventually, one evening in church at the beginning of 2002, as we were singing a song that says "My pain is healed in His name" I thought, What kind of a Christian woman am I if I can't have faith that God can heal me? So, I prayed that by whatever means necessary God would help me to find health again. The very next week my mother gave me her copy of the book The Natural Way. She had been offering it to me for a while and she and my father had changed their lifestyles with great results, but in the past I had just thought, How can changing the way I eat improve my health? Let me just say that until that point I ate reasonably healthy—only one piece of chocolate per month, only herbal tea, at least one fruit per day, good homemade pasta, fast food only once a week—I thought these were very healthy eating habits.

Needless to say after reading the book I decided I had nothing to lose. After two days my chest pains were gone, my stomach was not bloated, the flatulence stopped immediately, and I genuinely had energy for the first time in a very long time. I also began to notice an improvement in my concentration levels and memory. Even my reflexes improved. After about a month I began to lose weight, I could far exceed my previous level at the gym, and I battled to fall asleep at night due to the excessive energy I had. My depression lifted and I began to enjoy life again. I have not had another candida infection since. Now a year after starting with this correct eating plan—which is a lifestyle, not a diet—I am still experiencing all these benefits and can honestly say I will never go back. Thank you, Mary-Ann, for sharing your story, which has helped so many others, and thank you Lord for bringing this information across my path. God is good! I am so enthusiastic, in fact, that I am about to enroll in your nutritional course so that I can help others in the same boat as I.
Nereen

(Nereen now helps other people take responsibility for their health.)

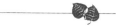

Hi Mary-Ann,
I was diagnosed in December 2003 as being osteopenic (just a hop and a skip away from osteoporosis) and I'm only forty-five. There was already an increased risk of bone fracture! I had the bone density scan done for fun! But I didn't think the result was such fun, and I took myself off to the doctor to see what now?

After a very thorough history taken by the GP, and after an expensive round of blood tests, the results came back that I'm genetically predisposed to osteoporosis! Nice one. The GP was a little worried because although I am short in stature that was the only "risk" factor I had for osteo. I don't smoke or drink, nor am I underweight. I was not on medication of any kind. The GP asked if I'd like to be referred to a physician. I replied that I saw little benefit in that. I asked her if my lifestyle could be to blame and she said "Yes, definitely."

So I decided to take responsibility for my health at long last. The mindset change of gaining health rather than losing weight was mind-

blowing for me. I was able to change my attitude radically and gave myself a year to get healthy. I follow the principles of the Natural Way and also started walking. (I'd been doing absolutely no exercise at that point due to many reasons that are not important right now.)

I have built up to walking about four miles at least six days a week and enjoy it now. I feel so good after walking. I have also lost 50 pounds in the process of gaining health and my Body Mass Index has changed from 30.7 to 22.4! I am feeling like a million dollars and looking great, too. I have more confidence and am determined to maintain my health plan. I do take barley grass juice and flaxseed oil daily. I am due to have another bone scan this coming December but it will be of academic interest as I am 100 percent convinced that there will be a change for the good in the result.

I wanted to share with you what exciting things have been happening in my life this year. And it's due to God giving me the strength to change my mindset regarding my health and following good eating principles that I've known about for ages but chose to ignore up until now.

Thank you, Mary-Ann, for caring enough to share your knowledge with so many others. I'm sure what you do is God's will for you.
Regards,
Sally

My journey on Perfect Health:
On June 30, 1988, I had a serious car accident in Johannesburg in which I sustained multiple injuries. After a month in the trauma unit I began the long process of rehabilitation. To compound my problems, the surgeons had missed a fracture of the acetabulum (hip socket) that had re-located while I was being pulled from the burning wreck. Many operations on the ruined hip joint ensued, resulting in permanent irreparable damage. I was on crutches for four years, until I was able to graduate to a walking stick, which I still use.

The prognosis was poor. Damage to the left leg was severe: bone and nerve damage, muscle wasting, and a substantial shortening. I was informed that I would be so immobile and in such pain within ten years that I would need major reconstructive surgery and would probably be on painkillers for the rest of my days. They also forecasted hip-replacement surgery every ten years after reconstruction, the success of which they couldn't guarantee anyway. Best advice: leave it alone until there was no other option; in other words, until I was completely immobile, or in unbearable pain.

I had nonetheless begun physiotherapy to make the best of a bad job, and one morning as I sat in my car, hung-over and finishing a cigarette, I heard this woman on the radio talking the most sense I had ever heard on the subject of nutrition and health. It was of course you, Mary-Ann. It all sounded so simple and logical that I just knew it had to be true. I got to know you and Mark and was soon following Perfect Health. My detox was quite severe given a combination of my previous lifestyle, numerous recent general anesthetics, and of course bucket-loads of medications.

Six months later, crutches and all, I was in the best shape of my life. People, including myself, were amazed at the transformation. I remember during an early morning breakfast function for a live Grammy Awards transmission, I was munching on fruit and watching people tuck into champagne and a greasy fry-up. I felt no desire to eat that kind of food any longer and was quite content to breakfast on fruit, feeling on top of the world. I've never forgotten how good I felt that morning.

In the intervening fifteen years I have strayed sometimes from Perfect Health, but have always come back. It has become a fundamental reference point in my life. I'm always grateful to come back to the Natural Way of life, and I always wonder why I strayed in the first place. Life is just so much better and enjoyable when you feel fit and healthy. Feeling fully alive is its own reward.

Oh, and by the way, I haven't taken a single painkiller for my leg in fifteen years, despite the dire predictions, and I am as mobile and active as I could ever have hoped to be given the permanent nature of my injury. Coincidence? I don't think so.
Robin Clark

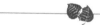

Dear Mark and Mary-Ann,
I have known you for years although you don't know me. I have attended some of your talks and read your book The Natural Way, *which is fading and tattered as this is my food bible.*

One tends to go off the path, which I have done feeling depressed and missing my family after I moved away. This resulted in headaches, ulcer pain, stomach cramps, and just feeling plain miserable. Funny enough I have your food-combining charts pinned inside my kitchen cupboard but didn't look at them for months. Then last week, after thinking I was dying from some unknown illness, the light bulb came on again and, voilà, both my husband and I are feeling wonderful. What a little effort for such great, astounding results! It is summer here in California so some days we just eat fruit all day. When I met my husband he was the typical American: fast-food and junk-food addict. Now he is studying the food-combination chart to make up the grocery list and hits the fruit stands first—it is actually quite hilarious. He lost 10 pounds just this last week and I lost 31 pounds, which is more than enough as I only weigh 122 pounds now.

I cannot tell you how wonderful I am feeling this morning—and just after a week of changing our food habits. Keep up the excellent work—you are an inspiration!

Regards,

Desiree

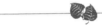

I am a Registered General, Psychiatric, and Community Nurse, as well as a Registered Midwife, and so I have a background in health-care. I have never been fully satisfied with the medical solutions offered to my patients, and although I admit that today's medicine does have its place, so many are not willing to learn that the body can heal itself. A friend introduced me to Perfect Health a few years back, and in preparation for a grueling and physically demanding hike I was to embark on six months from then, I decided to get myself into shape following the guidelines set out in Perfect health.

I subsequently lost 45 pounds, and have never looked or felt healthier in my life. Of course I was younger and did not have any physical ailments at the time, but I could see the difference in skin tone and my fitness and energy levels soared. I also suffered from mild depression, which disappeared completely.

I flew through the hike over six days in the mountains, but as soon as we got back to Cape Town, the fun began and the Natural Way flew out the window.

A while ago I decided that it was time to take control once again, as I have a family now (and you know what can happen to a person's body after a pregnancy). The energy and health natural to all of us is essential for living life to the fullest, whether it be work, play, or creating a better future.

It went slowly, but I realized that the weight I was carrying couldn't come off in a week. The mild depression and body aches and pains I lived with for so long have completely disappeared! A person has to remember each day that 1) everything happens in its time, 2) nobody can change overnight, and 3) every little improvement counts! We are all human, but ultimately capable of so much. I have studied anatomy and physiology but a person can never study the power of the body to recover—it has to be seen to be believed. After all, the One who created us knew what He was doing! All we have to do is treat ourselves with a little respect—the body does the rest.

Thank you,

Kay

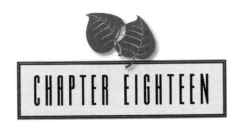

CHAPTER EIGHTEEN

Cooking Up a Storm
The Natural Way

ALL THE RECIPES in this chapter are suitable for a family of four to five with large appetites. We enjoy our food and are particularly fond of Italian dishes, with Mark loving his curry and chili dishes. These meals are intended to be quick and easy, as well as tasty and healthy. Any of the ingredients can be left out, or increased or decreased—just adapt the recipes to your family's taste, lifestyle, and pocket. It is important to note that these are by no stretch of the imagination gourmet meals. The idea behind them is to have fun and to enjoy cooking healthy food. Anyone in the family should be able to prepare these dishes. Mark and our girls were able to make all these meals, and they often did. The girls are now grown up and are in huge demand by friends as they are of the minority that can actually cook, and their friends love the healthy meals they make.

I have divided the recipes into the five steps to make following them easier for you. Then they are divided into neutral, starch, and protein sections to make choosing a properly combined meal easy. Neutral dishes can be served either with starch or protein, or they can be enjoyed on their own. Starch dishes should be served with a salad and combined well with any neutral vegetables. Protein dishes combine well with salads and neutral vegetables, but not with starches.

I have deliberately kept the protein section small as any animal protein should be cooked as simply as possible, either grilled or roasted and preferably without added fat. Thin slivers of fish, chicken, or meat can be added to any neutral dish, including the salads, to make a protein meal. Remember, there is no physiological reason to eat animal flesh.

When cooking Perfect Health meals, you will find that you spend far less time in the kitchen, and that you enjoy your time there far more. Enjoy the foods God created by doing as little to them as possible. Remember to keep the dishes simple and to start each cooked, non-fruit meal with raw vegetables. (For more recipes see www.mary-anns.com and subscribe to the monthly Digimag, which is a DVD showing us making various dishes plus other topics of interest. Look out for the *Perfect Health Recipe Book*.)

If you have any difficulty finding any of the ingredients or utensils mentioned in the book, please feel free to contact us at www.mary-anns. com. We also sell the Mary-Ann's seasonings that are mentioned in some of the recipes. For a detailed day-by-day program with recipes go to www.100daystohealth.com

Good luck and enjoy yourself!

Step 1: Eat One Fruit Meal a Day

The best way to eat any fruit is in its whole state, but to make your fruit meals a bit more interesting you might like to try some of these suggestions. Remember to buy fruit in season. Not only are they cheaper, but they taste far nicer, too. Summer fruits include mangoes, litchis, grapes, watermelons, peaches, nectarines, apricots, cherries, strawberries, and plums, while the winter fruits are oranges, tangerines, papaya, kiwi, guavas, apples, and pears. Although many of these fruits are available all year round, they are often kept in cold storage for up to nine months. Oranges and apples in particular are stored in this way. Flavor and nutrients are lost during storage and the cores are often bad. Bananas and pineapple are available all year round.

IDEAS FOR BLENDED FRUIT SHAKES OR SMOOTHIES

Blended shakes are a delicious and easy way to get reluctant fruit-eaters to turn to fruit with relish. Remember that although the fruits are blended and served in a glass, these shakes are a food and should be sipped slowly.

Some ideas:

Mango and pineapple (add a couple of passion fruit if you wish)
Mango and nectarine
Mango and peach
Papaya, banana, and dates
Mango and banana
Pineapple and strawberry or any berry for that matter

In fact, if you blend any of the sub-acid fruits with acid fruits, or any sub-acid fruits with sweet fruits, you are sure to have a delicious fruit shake. The same principle applies to fruit salad combinations. Here you could add some dates, raisins, or sultanas to any sweet fruit combination.

The acid and sub-acid combinations can have a quarter to half a cup of raw nuts or seeds added to make them more nutritious and help sustain your blood sugar longer.

Frozen fruits may be used as long as they contain no preservatives.

FROZEN STRAWBERRY AND PINEAPPLE COOLER

2 cups frozen strawberries (or other berries)
1 large pineapple
Raw honey, to taste

Strawberries have an anti-viral effect and help prevent heart disease and cancer due to their powerful antioxidant properties. Strawberries appear to block one of the most powerful cancer-forming substances, nitrosamines. They are also high in pectin, a water-soluble fiber that helps reduce cholesterol significantly.

They are also high in polyphenols, powerful antioxidants. People who eat strawberries regularly are three times less likely to get cancer than those who don't eat strawberries.

FROZEN FRUIT POPSICLES

Blend together a variety of fruit mixes and freeze in popsicle molds:

2 cups strawberries
½ cup passion fruit pulp
2 teaspoons orange rind

1 pineapple
2 mangoes

3 mangoes
½ cup passion fruit pulp

*Overripe bananas—place ½ banana
on a popsicle stick and freeze*

Any fresh fruit juice or blended fruit (kiwi is especially good)

Bananas are best peeled and placed whole in a plastic bag and frozen overnight. The next day, blend in a food processor and scoop into a bowl like "soft serve". All these frozen fruit pops are delicious and will satisfy any child's craving for ice cream. They have the additional advantage of being sugar- and dairy-free; they are loaded with nutrients and are alkaline in the bloodstream.

CASHEW OR ALMOND SHAKE

¼ cup cashews (or almonds) per person
¼–½ pineapple per person
¼–½ cup fresh orange or apple juice per person
Strawberries or passion fruit optional

Place all ingredients in a blender and blend until very smooth and creamy.

Tip: add ice cubes after blending the nuts and the shake gets very white and frothy.

Add less juice to make a thick cream and serve on a mixed acid/sub-acid fruit salad. You may prefer to add the passion fruit pulp last and just stir to prevent the gritty pieces from the seeds being chopped.

You can also extract the juice of fresh fruit if you are in a hurry and eat a handful of nuts afterward. Here is one of my favorite juices but you can combine any that you like.

GREEN BOOSTER

4 Granny Smith apples
½ pineapple
3 pears
1 lemon
Large piece ginger
Big bunch parsley

Extract the juice of the ingredients above and serve chilled with ice.

Apples are an excellent source of pectin, a water-soluble fiber that helps protect you from heart disease as it helps lower cholesterol and blood pressure. It also stabilizes blood sugar, keeping your appetite under control. Apple juice has been found to be antiviral and antibacterial and contains caffeic or chlorgenic acid, which is believed to prevent cancer formation at the cellular level.

Ginger helps with nausea, thins blood, lowers blood cholesterol, and has been shown to prevent cancer.

Pears are high in potassium and magnesium, both nutrients that help you relax and are highly alkaline.

Pineapple contains an enzyme called bromeline that aids digestion; it is high in natural vitamin C, a powerful antioxidant known to boost the immune system and slow down aging.

Parsley is part of the green leafy family and very high in chlorophyll, which is known to improve immune function.

Step 2: Snack on Raw Fruit or Vegetables or Nuts or Seeds Before You Eat Refined Sugar or Heated Fats

Together with Step 3

Step 2: Start All Cooked Meals with Raw Vegetables

A great way to start your meals is with either a salad or raw vegetable crudités (sticks). To help make this more enjoyable include a dip for the vegetables.

If you are not in the mood for making a salad you can also drink a glass of freshly extracted vegetable juice.

TOMATO AND RED PEPPER SMOOTHIE

2–3 large ripe tomatoes, seeds removed
2–3 large red bell peppers, seeds removed

Place in blender; blend with 1–2 cups ice cubes until smooth, season to suit palate with Mary-Ann's Organic Herb Salt, other herbal salt, juice a few celery sticks for a totally natural flavor, or pass through a juice extractor for a juice.

Serve garnished with fresh basil leaves.

CARROT, CELERY, AND TOMATO JUICE

For each person take the following and extract the juice in a juice extractor:

5 carrots
2 tomatoes
1–2 sticks celery

Celery is highly alkaline-forming and naturally high in sodium (an alkaline mineral), which adds flavor to savory dishes.

DIPS FOR RAW VEGETABLES

GUACAMOLE

4 avocados
2–3 spring onions or shallots, finely chopped
1 medium zucchini
½ cup cilantro (coriander) leaves
1–2 fresh green chilies, puréed (include seeds if you like it very hot)
Juice of ½ a lemon
1–2 teaspoons Mary-Ann's Organic Garlic & Herb Salt
or other herbal salt, to taste

Blend all ingredients well and serve with raw vegetables or as a topping for any meal.

CASHEW & OLIVE PASTE

1 cup cashews
12–15 black olives, pits removed

Blend together well until smooth and add a little fresh lemon juice and water if a creamier consistency is needed.

SUN-DRIED TOMATO PESTO

1 cup sun-dried tomatoes (must be free of sulfur dioxide)
½ cup cold-pressed extra-virgin olive oil
1 teaspoon Mary-Ann's Organic Garlic & Herb Salt
or other herbal salt
2 teaspoons dried basil or a handful of fresh basil leaves
1 tablespoon fresh (or 1 teaspoon dried) oregano
1 cup tomato purée

Soften the tomatoes in a little warm water, drain and place in a blender with the other ingredients, and blend until smooth; store in a jar in the refrigerator. Add a chili or two if you like a bit of heat.

QUICK HUMMUS

1 can garbanzo beans, drained
About 3–4 tablespoons extra-virgin olive oil
Mary-Ann's Organic Garlic & Herb Salt, to taste
Juice of 1 lemon
1 teaspoon cumin, ground
½ cup tahini (sesame seed paste)
½ cup filtered water
1 chili(optional)

Blend the beans with the lemon juice, water, and spices until smooth
and then add the tahini last, adding extra water if too thick; taste to
adjust seasoning and serve with raw vegetables.

MEXICAN BEAN DIP

2 cups cooked beans (or 1 can drained)—red beans
are best but any type is okay
¼ cup tomato purée (sugar-free)
1–2 teaspoons Mary-Ann's Organic Garlic & Herb Salt
1–2 whole medium chilies (optional)
Juice of ½ a lemon
1 teaspoon dried (or 1 tablespoon fresh) basil
2 spring onions or shallots
1–2 celery stalks

Blend all ingredients until fine. You can add a little olive oil to this
as well. Serve as a dip or a spread.

AUBERGINE (EGGPLANT) PÂTÉ

2 large eggplants (also known as aubergines in Europe)
Juice of 1 lemon
3 tablespoons extra-virgin olive oil
Mary-Ann's Organic Herb Salt or other herbal salt, to taste
2 tablespoons chopped parsley
1 bunch spring onions (optional)

Bake the aubergines in a medium oven at 320°F for 45 minutes. Peel off the skin and squeeze off any excess juice. Place in a food processor and blend with half the lemon juice and the onions. Add one tablespoon of oil. With the blender running, add the rest of the oil, the salt, and the remaining lemon juice. Add the parsley, spin once, and pour into a bowl and chill. Serve with raw vegetables.

SALADS

A fresh raw salad can be eaten before meals in place of raw vegetables and dip; Salads should be fun, tasty, and easy to prepare. At a restaurant, order a salad before the main course as your starter. If there is another cooked starter on the menu that you would like, have it either with your main meal or as your main meal.

Here I refer specifically to fresh salad, not cooked salads. If there are cooked ingredients such as artichokes or garbanzo beans, try to add as many other raw ingredients as possible. In our family, avocados are a staple salad ingredient. But avocados are a much-maligned fruit. Mention that you eat avocados and people throw up their hands in horror with shrieks of "fattening" and "cholesterol." Let's get one thing straight: there is not a single fruit or vegetable that is able to manufacture cholesterol—this process is confined to the animal kingdom (see chapter eight). Although avocados do contain fats, they are unsaturated fats that are easy to digest and contain essential fatty acids that help the hormonal system to function properly and can actually help you lose weight.

Avocados are also extremely nutritious, containing fourteen minerals, eleven vitamins, and a high percentage of protein for a fruit. (Yes, avocado is a fruit although we do tend to eat it as a vegetable.)

Avocados are in season from autumn through winter to the following mid-summer, which means that they are unobtainable for three or four months of the year only. I might add that this short period of deprivation makes Mark's life a misery. He can't bear salad without avocado and insists on adding olives or cheese to make it more interesting. The olives are not a problem but regular cheese results in him snoring at night so to keep the cheese to a minimum I usually make marinated mushrooms or eggplant (see recipes). Mark's favorite way of eating avocados is to have them mashed on hot, buttered toast. I like to use avocados as a skin treatment—I use the inside of the skin to rub on my hands. It is the most wonderful skin cream and has the added benefit of being completely natural and additive-free.

A word of caution—if you want to lose weight, don't eat more than one avocado per day. If, on the other hand, you are trying to gain some weight, try to eat at least three avocados every day.

Here is a recipe for our favorite salad (which contains avocado, of course). We adapt it in a number of ways and I have included the variations below.

BASIC AVOCADO SALAD

1 medium lettuce, broken into bite-sized pieces
4 medium tomatoes, sliced or diced
4 medium avocados, diced
1 red bell pepper, sliced or chopped
2 sticks celery, chopped
1 tablespoon parsley, chopped (optional)
2 carrots, cut into small strips
Mary-Ann's Organic Herb Salt or other herbal salt, to taste

Toss all the ingredients together in a large salad bowl and serve. The avocado makes this salad deliciously creamy. Add a bit of herbal salt and pepper to taste if you like. This salad can be served with either a protein or a starch meal, or inside whole wheat pita bread.

Variations on a Theme

Any of the following ingredients can be added to the Basic Avocado Salad:

Olives in brine (not vinegar)
Asparagus tips, fresh or canned
Thin slices of chicken or other meat
Flaked tuna
Feta cheese
Cubed uncolored cheese
Red cabbage, chopped

Special note: if you add cheese, chicken, fish, or meat to the salad, it is no longer a neutral dish but becomes a protein meal.

AVOCADO STARTERS

For a delicious and healthy start to any meal, serve avocado in the shell. Allow half an avocado per person, remove the pit, and rub the flesh with lemon juice to prevent discoloration. Fill with any of the following mixtures:

Add homemade mayonnaise to:

Chopped chicken, chopped spring onions,
sliced mushrooms, Mary-Ann's Organic Herb Salt,
pepper, and lemon juice (protein meal)

Asparagus pieces with chopped olives (neutral meal)

Grated uncolored cheese and chopped spring onions
(protein or neutral meal depending on which cheese you use)

Add ricotta cheese (ricotta cheese is low in protein—less than 15 percent—so these salads are neutral unless animal flesh is added, although can still cause mucus problems) to:

Chopped red pepper and olives

Chopped cucumber and celery seasoned with Mary-Ann's
Organic Herb Salt or Seasoning Salt

Add sour cream (sour cream is neutral as it is low in protein, but it is a fat so use sparingly) to:

Flaked tuna, chopped chives, and lemon juice

Chopped tomato, fresh basil, and spring onions

Cucumber

Another way to serve the avocado would be to mash the flesh with any of the above fillings and to return the mixture to the shell, or to spoon it onto a lettuce leaf.

Special note: try to eat only those vegetables that are in season. They are cheaper and tastier. Any good gardening book on vegetables will be able to tell you which vegetables are in season.

AVOCADO SAUCES, DRESSINGS, AND DIPS

Avocado dips are a particularly good way of getting children to eat salad as they are often not all that fond of raw vegetables. Make up a platter of sliced raw vegetables—such as cucumber, celery, zucchini, steamed asparagus, carrots, tomatoes, red pepper, or broccoli and cauliflower (either raw or lightly steamed)—and serve with one of the following dips:

Avocado, tomato, and fresh basil
Avocado, tomato, red pepper, and celery
Avocado, sour cream, fresh lemon juice, and herbal salt
Avocado, black pepper, and chopped chives
Avocado, lemon juice, herbal salt, and pepper

Blend the ingredients in a food processor and add a little filtered water if a more fluid salad dressing is required. The quantities and proportions of ingredients depend on your personal preferences. The blended dips (without additional water) are also suitable as sauces for dressing steamed vegetables, chicken, or fish.

ASPARAGUS AND AVOCADO SALAD

1. Gently steam 1–2 bunches of fresh asparagus, until bright green.
2. Place 3–5 pieces of asparagus on each plate.
3. Place ½ a sliced avocado on each of the plates of asparagus.
4. Squeeze a little fresh lemon juice over the avocado.
5. Sprinkle freshly chopped parsley, cilantro, or rocket.
6. Drizzle with Red Pepper Mayonnaise (see below) and serve.

RED PEPPER MAYONNAISE

3–4 medium red bell peppers
½ cup cold-pressed olive oil
Juice of 1 lemon
1 teaspoon oregano
Mary-Ann's Organic Garlic & Herb Salt or other herbal salt, to taste

Coarsely chop the peppers and place in a small pot. Simmer gently with a lid on for about 15 minutes. Drain the juices well. Purée well in a food processor and add the oil drop by drop, add the rest of the ingredients, and blend well. Adjust the salt for taste and serve.

MARINATED MUSHROOMS

2 cups white mushrooms, thinly sliced
1 cup extra-virgin olive oil
1–2 teaspoons ready-prepared mustard or mustard seeds
½ cup parsley, chopped
1 teaspoon Mary-Ann's Organic Seasoning Salt
or Herb Salt with a pinch of nutmeg
Juice of 1 lemon

Blend all the ingredients by hand and place the mushrooms in the marinade for at least 30 minutes. Button and brown mushrooms give a very different flavor so try them both.

Serve on sliced avocado or just plain lettuce leaves or any salad that needs a "pick-me-up."

ROASTED RED PEPPER AND ARTICHOKE SALAD

½–1 lettuce with red leaves (Lollo Rosso)
½–1 head butter or crisp lettuce
5–10 continental spinach leaves
2 red peppers
5–6 artichoke hearts, drained and quartered
¼–½ cup raw nuts, such as hazelnuts, cashews, or almonds
3 ounces Gorgonzola or blue cheese

Clean the peppers, cut them into eighths, and roast gently on a baking sheet, without using oil.

Arrange the artichokes and red peppers on a bed of lettuce leaves. Sprinkle with nuts and crumbled cheese. Drizzle with extra-virgin, 100%-pure cold-pressed olive oil; add a dash of freshly squeezed lemon juice or balsamic vinegar, a twist of the pepper grinder, and herbal salt to taste.

GARBANZO, AVOCADO, AND CABBAGE SALAD

3 cups cabbage, finely shredded
1 can garbanzo beans, drained
2–3 avocados, diced
Juice of 1 small lemon
Black olives (optional)
Fresh or preservative-free sun-dried tomatoes (soaked to soften),
or 1–2 cups cubed tomatoes or red bell peppers
Mary-Ann's Organic Seasoning Salt

Combine gently so as not to mash the avocado. (Mark and I often eat this as a meal because it is so filling.)

Garbanzo beans are part of the bean family and are known to reduce bad LDL cholesterol. They contain protease inhibitors known to inhibit cancer, regulate blood sugar and insulin—type 2 diabetics have been shown to eliminate the need for medication by eating them daily—lower blood pressure, regulate colon function, prevent and correct constipation, and prevent hemorrhoids and other bowel problems. All beans contain a glucose called alpha-galactose that can cause gas but within a few days of eating regularly you will produce the enzymes needed to digest this.

Olives and olive oil have been shown to be good for the heart, reduce bad cholesterol, raise good cholesterol, thin blood, and contain phytonutrients that retard cancer and aging, increase longevity, and lower blood pressure.

SALAD WITH VEGETABLE CROUTONS

2 eggplants, diced or cubed
4–6 zucchini, diced (and/or carrots, beets, potatoes)

Place on baking tray and sprinkle with herbal salt. Bake at a hot temperature or on grill until golden brown; remove and cool.

Combine with the following:

Mixed lettuce
3–4 tomatoes, chopped
2 avocados, diced

Serve with extra-virgin olive and/or flaxseed oil, juice of ½–1 lemon, Mary-Ann's Organic Herb Salt, and freshly ground black pepper.

STEAMED BROCCOLI & AVOCADO SALAD

1. Cut 2 cups broccoli into bite-sized pieces and lightly steam.
2. Squeeze juice of 1 lemon over broccoli and season with Mary-Ann's Organic Seasoning Salt or herbal salt with pepper and a pinch of nutmeg.
3. Serve garnished with lots of cubed or sliced avocados.
4. Add chopped red peppers and/or sun-dried tomatoes.
5. Optional: include steamed, sliced brown mushrooms.

Broccoli is part of the cruciferous family and as such is very high in the anti-cancer substances known as indoles, glucosinolates, and dihiolthiones, which are known to actually help the body destroy cancer cells.

ROCKET (ARUGULA) SALAD

2–4 cups small white mushrooms (whole if small, halved if large)
1 red bell pepper, sliced
1 yellow bell pepper, sliced
10 black olives in brine (not vinegar or oil)
½ cup cold-pressed extra-virgin olive oil
Mary-Ann's Organic Garlic & Herb Salt, to taste
1 tablespoon lemon juice
2 large handfuls of rocket or other green leaves of your choice

Blend the oil, salt, and lemon juice and pour over mushrooms and peppers. Allow to marinate for at least 10 minutes.

Pour over leaves and garnish with olives.

Red and yellow bell peppers are ripe and easy to digest (unlike green) and they are high in antioxidants such as vitamin C and beta carotene, which have a powerful effect on the immune system and slow down aging.

Mushrooms thin blood, prevent cancer, lower blood cholesterol, and stimulate the immune system by encouraging the body to produce more interferon (lentinan—a long chain sugar), inactivating viruses.

SAUCES AND DRESSINGS

Our favorite salad dressing is an avocado dressing, which is really just one of the dips in the salad section. We add either a little more lemon juice to thin it out, or a little filtered water. You might like to try some of our other favorites—they enhance a wide variety of salads.

OLIVE AND LEMON DRESSING

1 cup extra-virgin olive oil
Juice of 1 lemon
1 teaspoon Mary-Ann's Organic Herb Salt or other herbal salt
Freshly ground black pepper
1–2 teaspoons fresh mixed herbs, chopped
(oregano, thyme, and basil are good)

Place all the ingredients in a closed jar or container. Shake well and serve immediately or store in the fridge.

HOMEMADE MAYONNAISE

This mayonnaise can be eaten with starch or protein as egg yolks are very low in protein.

2 organic egg yolks
1 teaspoon dry mustard
½ teaspoon Mary-Ann's Organic Herb Salt, Garlic and Herb Salt, or other herbal salt
Freshly ground black pepper
Juice of 1 lemon
1 cup cold-pressed olive, flaxseed, or a blend of extra-virgin oils
Dash cayenne pepper (optional)

Place the egg yolks in a blender with the dry ingredients and blend well using the steel blade. Add the lemon juice slowly, using the pulse button. Add the oil in a very slow stream while the blender is running. A teaspoon of boiling water can be added to thin the mayonnaise if necessary.

Tip: the egg yolks must be at room temperature and the oil must be added very slowly. The blender must be running the entire time.

SOME QUICK DRESSINGS (NEUTRAL)

- Melted butter and lemon juice are good when poured over any lightly steamed vegetables, grilled chicken, or fish. They are particularly delicious over broccoli and zucchini
- Freshly squeezed lemon juice can be drizzled over fresh salads with extra-virgin olive and/or flaxseed oil
- Blended tomato, basil, Mary-Ann's Organic Herb Salt, pepper, and a little oil (optional) is a good dressing for salads, vegetables, or your favorite pasta

NEUTRAL DISHES

These dishes should be served either with a protein or a starch, or they can be enjoyed on their own. They are alkaline-forming and it would be best to have bigger portions of cooked neutral vegetables than starches or proteins.

VEGETABLES

Vegetables are generally at their nicest in winter, especially potatoes, butternut squash, broccoli, cauliflower, and Brussels sprouts. Avocados are abundant in the winter and are very reasonably priced at this time of year. Vegetables are best eaten raw or lightly steamed. A stainless steel retractable steamer or a bamboo steamer is particularly efficient. The next best are frozen vegetables, followed by additive-free canned varieties, although I rarely use canned artichokes, asparagus, and garbanzo beans as canned food is cooked at high temperatures. As dried vegetables are usually treated with sulfur dioxide, it is best to avoid them.

Some Quick Ideas

- Take 2 cups of broccoli and 1 small cauliflower, cut into small sprigs and steam for 5–10 minutes. Arrange in a dish in rings of contrasting colors. Dot with butter and squeeze some fresh lemon juice over the florets. Steamed button mushrooms added to this are also very tasty, and an avocado dressing makes the dish something special

- Steamed fresh asparagus rolled in butter and drizzled with lemon juice is delicious, or served with homemade mayonnaise
- Brussels sprouts or fresh broccoli steamed and served with butter and chopped mint or flaked almonds are a treat
- Fresh garden peas steamed and dotted with butter are good with chopped mint
- Baby carrots (or julienne slices) steamed and tossed with chopped parsley and butter are very tasty
- Thinly sliced zucchini steamed with button mushrooms and tossed in butter are always popular
- Steamed broccoli tossed together with button mushrooms, diced avocado, and sliced rings of red pepper make an unusual and delicious dish
- Steamed spinach blended in a food processor with fresh cream, herbal salt, and black pepper make an excellent—feta cheese can be used instead of the cream
- Steamed button mushrooms and baby corn are another favorite
- Make a quick and delicious casserole by cutting a wide variety of seasonal vegetables into bite-size pieces and placing them in an ovenproof dish with 2–3 teaspoons organic or 100% natural vegetable stock and a little filtered water. Cover the dish and bake at 356°F for 50 minutes
- Bake whole butternut squash at 320°F–356°F for an hour. When done, cut the butternut in half lengthways and scoop out the pits. Serve with pats of butter or stuff with brown rice or a vegetable mixture or tomato pesto (add a chili if you like) and a little sour cream

VEGETABLE SOUP

Place any and as many different sorts of vegetables in a large pot and cover with 1–2 liters of water. Add 1–2 teaspoons of MSG-free vegetable stock powder or cubes for flavor. Season with Mary-Ann's Organic Herb Salt; potatoes or barley can be added, but bear in mind that the soup then becomes a starch meal.

Special note: when serving soup, do not forget to start with some raw vegetables. Remember that soup is a food and that it should be chewed or swirled in the mouth, not just gulped down.

MUSHROOM SOUP

1 small bunch spring onions, finely chopped
1 medium carrot, sliced
1 celery stalk, sliced
2 cups white mushrooms, sliced
2–3 cups filtered water
Mary-Ann's Organic Seasoning Salt or pinch of nutmeg and herbal salt
4 tablespoons thick cream

Dry stir-fry (see below) chopped onions, gently stirring the entire time over medium heat. Add the carrot, celery, and mushrooms to stir-fry. Add the water and simmer gently for about 15 minutes. Add seasoning and serve. Alternatively blend in a food processor, reheat, and add the cream while sprinkling the nutmeg. This soup can be served with a salad and whole wheat bread as a starch meal, or with salad and a protein.

Dry stir-frying is just stir-frying without any oil or fat. You stir quickly over a medium to high heat and add the oil, butter, or cream just before serving. This makes the meal more digestible as heated fats are difficult to digest and can promote cancer and prostate problems.

QUICK BEST EVER TOMATO SOUP

12–15 very ripe tomatoes
2 sweet potatoes or yams
6 carrots
Mary-Ann's Organic Garlic & Herb Salt
2–4 teaspoons natural vegetable stock (MSG-free)
Fresh basil
Olive oil, to taste
Mary-Ann's Organic Seasoning Salt or herbal salt and a pinch of nutmeg
1 cup organic double thick cream

Chop the vegetables coarsely, then add and simmer gently until all are soft (about 1 hour).

Blend until smooth and serve with a swirl of olive oil (or organic fresh sour cream for special occasions) and fresh crusty homemade bread or rice cakes if gluten intolerant.

CREAMED SPINACH

1 bunch spinach, washed and chopped (remove coarse stalks only)

Place in a pot and simmer in own water until soft. Drain well and squeeze out excess water. Chop and add olive oil. Season with Mary-Ann's Organic Seasoning Salt or herbal salt and a pinch of nutmeg (the nutmeg lifts the spinach flavor). Blend well with the cream and serve.

For special occasions add a bit of feta cheese.

QUICK AND SIMPLE RATATOUILLE

1 onion, chopped (optional—I prefer celery)
3 eggplants, sliced or diced
2 cups zucchini, sliced
2 red bell peppers, sliced
2 cups mushrooms, sliced (optional)
4–5 large tomatoes, peeled and chopped
Fresh oregano, chopped to taste (dried is also fine)
Mary-Ann's Organic Herb Salt or other herbal salt, to taste

Layer the ingredients in a casserole dish or saucepan, and either bake at 392°F for 30 minutes to an hour, or simmer gently on the stove in a pot or saucepan.

Special note: as a variation, add a layer of sliced potato and make a starch meal of this dish.

ASPARAGUS WITH À LA KING SAUCE

4 cups of different variety mushrooms, sliced
2–4 cups asparagus pieces
1 tablespoon butter
1 heaped tablespoon whole wheat, pea, rice, corn, or potato flour
1 cup cream or soy milk
2 cups frozen peas

Stir-fry mushrooms over medium heat without water or oil. Add asparagus chunks (reserve juice), peas, butter, and enough flour to absorb the moisture. Add the asparagus juice from the can or filtered water, stirring the entire time. Add cream and heat through.

Serve dish on its own with a fresh salad to start or spoon over a bed of brown rice or noodles for a starch meal.

SAVORY MUSHROOMS

4–6 cups mushrooms (about 1 pound)
Extra-virgin olive oil or 2 teaspoons butter
Mary-Ann's Organic Seasoning Salt or Herb Salt
with a pinch of nutmeg and freshly ground pepper

Wash mushrooms carefully and place them whole in a small pot or medium saucepan. Sprinkle with seasoning salt, and simmer for 15–20 minutes. Serve as a main or side dish with a starch or protein and/or other vegetables. Drizzle with olive oil. Don't forget the salad.

MUSHROOMS FLORENTINE

1 large black mushroom per person (starter)
or
2–3 large black mushrooms per person (main course)
Creamed spinach (see earlier recipe)

Steam or grill the mushrooms lightly. Spoon creamed spinach on top of each mushroom and add a sprinkling of Parmesan or crumbled feta cheese or chopped cashews or almonds if you want a protein meal. Pop back under the grill and garnish with tomato slices.

This dish is a good starter with some raw salad, or a filling main course if served with a starch or protein.

ZUCCHINI & MUSHROOM BAKE

3–4 spring onions or shallots, finely chopped
2–4 cups large brown mushrooms, sliced
2 medium eggplants, thinly sliced and dry-grilled
until lightly browned
Mary-Ann's Organic Garlic & Herb Salt
2 tablespoons Parmesan cheese

1 teaspoon oregano
½ cup chopped parsley
Pinch thyme
1 cup tomato purée
1 cup fresh cream
4 cups zucchini, sliced into rounds
4–6 ripe tomatoes, sliced

Layer the mushrooms, spring onions, and eggplants, sprinkling the herbs and cheese in between. Pour over the cream and tomato pu-rée.

Arrange the zucchini and tomato slices on top, overlapping in rows. Sprinkle with parsley and thyme. Season with salt and freshly ground black pepper. Bake for 30–40 minutes at 356°F, remove, lightly sprinkle with Parmesan cheese, return and bake for another 15 minutes.

Step 4: Food-Combining: Keep Your Meals Simple by Eating Starches and Proteins at Separate Meals

STARCH DISHES

Starch dishes should be served with a salad and with any neutral veg-etable dish. They should never be served with a protein as this is a poor combination. Try not eating starch more than once a day if you want to lose weight.

GRILLED POLENTA TOWERS ON CREAMED SPINACH

1 slice of polenta per person
2 x ½ inch slices eggplant per person (seasoned with Mary-Ann's Organic Garlic & Herb Salt)
2 x ½ inch slices ripe tomato per person (seasoned with Mary-Ann's Organic Herb Salt)
1 cup creamed spinach per person

Lightly toast or grill the polenta in a hot oven until golden brown.

Bake or grill the tomato and eggplant slices in a hot oven until soft but not mushy. (The eggplant takes longer to cook.)

Cook polenta according to instructions on the packet. When ready, pour out on a tray or kitchen table and spread evenly until ½ inch thick; cool and cut into 3–4 inch square slices.

Place slices of polenta on a baking sheet and top each slice with a slice of grilled eggplant, a slice of tomato, a slice of grilled eggplant, one tomato, and a slice of mozzarella cheese. You can use a skewer to hold in place. Pop under the grill to heat through; place each slice on a bed of spinach and serve with fresh salad.

Spinach is a dark green leafy vegetable packed with nutrients; it is known to prevent cancer alongside carrots, specifically colon, rectal, stomach, prostate, laryngeal, endometrial, and lung cancers. Studies find that people who eat the least dark green leafy vegetables have the highest rates of cancer. (Sprouted barley leaves are the most nutritious of this family, one of the many reasons I advocate drinking barley grass juice.)

Consuming these dark green leafy vegetables increases your intake of 2'-0-Glycosylisovitexin and peroxides, found in extremely high, but safe levels and these together with enzymes called peroxides have been shown to be anti-carcinogenic and anti-mutagenic. Peroxides actually break down and neutralize Try-P1 and P2, carcinogens in grilled meat and fish, and 3-4benzypyrene, another carcinogen in tobacco.

Dark green leafy vegetables are our best sources of calcium. However, the oxalic acid in spinach binds the calcium in these leaves so don't rely on this as a source.

Corn (polenta) is high in protease inhibitors known to prevent cancer. It is best eaten unrefined and natural like polenta. The natural fat in corn or maize products is known to lower cholesterol. Corn is also believed to reduce the risk of tooth cavities. Polenta and fine corn grits are similar and can be used either way.

Eggplant is a good source of fiber and vitamin A, potassium, phosphorus, calcium, and small amounts of protein, and it protects arteries against cholesterol damage. It also prevents against cancer and contains chemicals that prevent convulsions.

Tomato is high in lycopene, part of the carotenoid family, and is also high in vitamin C. It also contains calcium (as does all plant food), magnesium, potassium, and is alkaline in your bloodstream when eaten raw; it is thought to be beneficial for liver and kidney problems and research indicates that it helps prevent cancer and appendicitis.

POTATO PANCAKES WITH HERBED TOMATOES

5 medium potatoes (pre-cooked)
¼–½ cup potato, corn, or whole wheat flour
(optional—I sometimes leave this out even though it crumbles a bit)
2 spring onions or shallots, finely chopped
¾ cup 100%-pure soymilk or fresh cream
1–2 teaspoons dried or fresh oregano
2 tablespoons extra-virgin cold-pressed olive oil
1 teaspoon Mary-Ann's Organic Seasoning Salt or salt, pepper,
and a pinch of nutmeg

Mash the potatoes, add the rest of the ingredients, and blend with a fork until well combined. Form into patties and bake in a hot oven (428–500°F) on a non-stick surface until golden brown.

HERBED TOMATOES

2–4 cups cherry tomatoes, cut into quarters
1 tablespoon fresh (or 2 teaspoons dried) oregano
½–1 cup pitted olives, sliced
4 spring onions, finely chopped
Mary-Ann's Organic Garlic & Herb Salt to taste

Bake in a separate dish (the potato pancakes go soggy if baked together) alongside the potatoes until hot and cooked. Drizzle with olive oil and serve on top of potato patties.

VEGETABLE CURRY

4 cups filtered water
6 teaspoons mixed curry powders (I have three different types
and use 2 teaspoons of each)
2 teaspoons ground cumin
1 teaspoon ground cinnamon
1 teaspoon ground turmeric
1 teaspoon ground ginger
1 teaspoon coarse salt
1 teaspoon ground coriander or a handful of fresh cilantro, chopped

½ *cup fresh lemon juice (optional)*
4–8 cups mixed fresh vegetables
2 fresh red medium chilies (optional if you want it hotter)

Place all the ingredients (except the vegetables) in a large pot and bring to a boil. Reduce heat and simmer for about 30 minutes. Add a combination of vegetables such as broccoli, green beans, carrots, and cauliflower, and simmer for another 30 minutes to 1 hour. If you want a butternut curry, use three large cubed butternuts instead of the mixed vegetables. Serve with brown rice.

Special note: this recipe is sufficient for 6 to 8 servings. It keeps well and is delicious if served at a later stage—the flavors seem to mature.

CUCUMBER RELISH (SERVED WITH CURRY)

1 English cucumber
1 tablespoon mint, chopped
1 red pepper, seeded and finely chopped
1 bunch spring onions, finely chopped
½ *cup sour cream*
1 teaspoon herbal salt
Pinch cayenne pepper

Grate the unpeeled cucumber and squeeze the excess water from the pulp in a sieve. Mix in the remaining ingredients, cover and chill until needed. Serve with a vegetable curry and rice.

BANANA RELISH (SERVED WITH CURRY)

4 ripe bananas
4 tablespoons sour cream
2 tablespoons honey

Mix the honey and sour cream well. When blended, pour over the bananas to coat. Serve immediately with vegetable curry and rice.

Special note: although it is not ideal to eat fruit with other foods, bananas or other sweet fruits can often be tolerated by the stomach when eaten with a starch. Do not, however, make a habit of this combination.

TOMATO AND ONION RELISH (SERVED WITH CURRY)

3 large ripe tomatoes, diced
3 bunches spring onions, chopped
3 teaspoons fresh lemon juice
Pinch cayenne pepper
1 teaspoon soy sauce (MSG-free)
½ teaspoon Mary-Ann's Organic Herb Salt

Mix all ingredients and chill until needed. Serve with a vegetable curry and brown rice.

WHEAT GERM STUFFING

A neutral stuffing eaten with protein like chicken, turkey, fish, or vegetables like baked potatoes:

4 heaped teaspoons wheat germ
2 tablespoons parsley, chopped
1 large, flat mushroom, finely chopped
1 tablespoon cold-pressed olive or sunflower oil
1 organic egg yolk
1 small bunch spring onions, chopped
1 teaspoon lemon juice
1 heaped teaspoon dried thyme
Pinch marjoram
Mary-Ann's Organic Seasoning Salt or Herb Salt and a pinch nutmeg
Salt and pepper

Mix all ingredients and adjust seasoning to taste. Mix with a little water to moisten (the stuffing must still be stiff though). Use as a stuffing for chicken or turkey and beef olives.

Special note: this is really delicious and no one would guess that wheat germ has been used instead of bread crumbs. As bread is a starch, it is not ideal for making stuffing for protein. Wheat germ is neutral and is suitable for any starch or protein combination.

VEGETABLE STUFFING

6 spring onions
2 sticks celery or shallots, finely chopped (I prefer
to use chopped celery)
2 teaspoons butter
2 cups button mushrooms, sliced
½–1 cup carrot, grated
1 tablespoon parsley, chopped
1 tablespoon pea, potato, or garbanzo bean flour
1 teaspoon dried mixed herbs
Mary-Ann's Organic Seasoning Salt or Herb Salt, pepper,
and a pinch of nutmeg

Dry stir-fry the onions in a pot. (To dry stir-fry just add ingredients to a hot pot and stir rapidly; you can add a little water if you prefer.) Add all the remaining ingredients except the flour. Cook until the water starts to draw and then add the flour. Cool and use to stuff a whole chicken, or alternatively, lift the skin off chicken pieces and fill with stuffing; dry roast the chicken in foil for 30 minutes at 392°F and then for another hour at 320°F. Serve with neutral vegetables and remember to start with a large salad.

Special note: this stuffing is also delicious in baked potatoes.

VEGETABLE STIR-FRY

1 cup onions, spring onions, or shallots, chopped
1 cup celery, chopped
1 cup carrots, coarsely grated
½ cup peas
½ cup green beans, sliced
1 cup cooked brown rice
1 tablespoon parsley, chopped
MSG-free soy sauce

Stir-fry the vegetables lightly in a little water, adding the mushrooms, parsley and soy sauce last. Add a pat of butter before serving. Start the meal with a large salad.

PERFECT MASHED POTATOES

1–2 large potatoes per person
Fresh thin cream or soy milk
Butter or extra-virgin olive oil
Mary-Ann's Organic Herb or Seasoning Salt

Steam the potatoes, unpeeled but chopped roughly, in a steamer or simmer gently in an inch of water. When done, mash (with the left-over water) with a fork or a potato masher. Believe it or not, the skins are quite delicious. The skins also encourage you to chew the potatoes and as you know, chewing gets the starch-digesting enzyme working. Add a little olive oil or butter, thin cream, and the salt.

Special note: mashed potatoes are even more delicious when you fold some lightly steamed mushrooms into the mixture. Mashed potatoes can also be piped over any vegetable casserole and baked in the oven, like cottage pie.

PERFECT BAKED POTATOES

Choose potatoes of equal size and wash well. Prick the skins with a fork to prevent the potatoes from bursting in the oven. Place on the oven rack and bake in a hot oven at 392°F for 50–60 minutes. When ready, remove from the oven and cut a deep cross in the center of each potato. Press the sides together gently to open the cross. Dot with butter or olive oil, add a dash of sour cream or cold-pressed olive oil, and sprinkle with chopped parsley. Baked potatoes are perfect for serving with a salad and any neutral vegetable.

Stuffing Baked Potatoes

Bake potatoes in the oven as above. When ready, slice the top off each potato, scoop out the flesh and mash with cold-pressed vege-table oil, butter, cream, or soy milk and a little Mary-Ann's Organic Herb or Seasoning Salt. Add steamed, sliced mushrooms and a dash of nutmeg to the mixture, or some chopped steamed spinach. Refill the skins, sprinkle with a little nutmeg, and return to a 392°F oven for 10 minutes, or until lightly brown.

Serve with a salad and any neutral vegetables.

POLENTA PIZZA

1. Place 3 cups water for every 1 cup polenta in a pot.
2. Bring to a boil and add ½ teaspoon sea salt per cup.
3. Stir in the polenta and turn the heat down to low. When they thicken place the lid on and then stir well every 10 minutes; if they become too thick add a little boiling water and stir to the consistency of thick porridge—in other words, keep their shape.
4. Remove from the pot and place on a large tray or a clean board or countertop. Flatten with a spatula to about ½ inch thick. Cool and cut into hand-sized squares. Spread with tomato pesto and top with any vegetable toppings and mozzarella cheese (if not dairy intolerant).
5. Bake in a hot oven until the edges crisp (be careful not to over-cook the cheese if using).
6. Optional: top with mashed avocado in place of cheese.

BAKED, FAT-FREE OVEN CHIPS

1. Slice 6–10 potatoes into chips or wedges. Leave the skins on, as they are more nutritious.
2. Place on a baking sheet and bake in a hot oven, at least 392°F for 45–60 minutes or until golden brown and soft when squeezed.
3. Remove and season with Mary-Ann's Organic Salts. I prefer my chips with extra-virgin olive oil, so add a drop or two, toss lightly, and serve (or without oil for the fat-free version).

MUSHROOM BURGER—PER PERSON

1 whole wheat or olive bread roll or two slices whole wheat bread
1 large brown mushroom (size of normal patty)
1–2 slices ripe tomatoes
1 lettuce leaf
A little chopped spring onion
Tomato pesto (see previous recipes)
Homemade mayonnaise (see previous recipes)
Cold-pressed extra-virgin olive oil or uncolored butter

Dry roast or grill the mushrooms by placing on an oven tray. Sprinkle with a little Mary-Ann's Seasoning Salt. This really lifts the taste of the mushroom. (Or add a pinch or nutmeg—be careful not to overdo it—and herb salt.) Place under the grill for 10–15 minutes and remove.

Drizzle the bread or roll with the olive oil or spread with butter.

Spread with tomato pesto, top with the mushroom, lettuce, spring onions, and tomato and drizzle with the mayonnaise.

Serve with baked chips.

POTATO CASSEROLE

2 medium potatoes per person
1 cup thin cream or soy milk
Salt and freshly ground black pepper
Spring onions, chopped (optional)
Mushrooms, sliced (optional)

Scrub potatoes thoroughly. Slice into ¼ inch slices. Layer potatoes (and onions and mushrooms if using) with seasoning and cream in an ovenproof dish and bake in a medium/hot oven at 356°F–392°F for about an hour. Although this dish is very simple, it is quite delicious. Remove the lid of the casserole dish halfway through for a crispy top.

MARK'S VEGETABLE CASSEROLE

1 red pepper, sliced or chopped
2 cups broccoli, cut into bite-sized pieces
1 packet baby corn, cut into bite-sized pieces
3–4 carrots, cut into strips
2 cups mushrooms
1 heaped teaspoon vegetable stock, dissolved in ½ cup hot water
½ cup soaked and strained lentils
2 teaspoons curry powder (optional) or a few extra chilies
1 can Italian tomato (optional)

Combine all ingredients in a casserole dish. Cover with lid and bake at 320°F–356°F (medium temperature) for an hour.

Mark came up with this recipe on a camping trip and it is delicious served on a bed of brown rice with a fresh green salad.

Special note: although canned food is not ideal, it can be used occasionally. Remember to go for only those brands free of artificial additives.

MUSHROOM STROGANOFF

1 pound ribbon noodles (rice noodles are especially good here)
4–6 cups mixed mushrooms, sliced
2–3 sticks celery or 3–4 shallots, chopped
1 cup sour cream
Mary-Ann's Organic Seasoning Salt or Herb Salt with a pinch nutmeg
and freshly ground black pepper

Cook noodles according to the instructions on the packet. Dry stir-fry the celery and the mushrooms in a little butter. Season and add the cream. Heat through and serve on top of the noodles.

Special note: on special occasions, sprinkle this dish with Parmesan or pecorino cheese and serve with homemade olive bread (see recipe for Never-Fail Whole Wheat Bread). The sauce can also be used with protein dishes or even with rice and potatoes.

ZUCCHINI RICE SALAD

3 cups cooked brown rice
2 cups zucchini, sliced and steamed
Mary-Ann's Organic Herb Salt
Ground black pepper, to taste
1 tablespoon fresh basil, chopped
1 red bell pepper, chopped
2–3 sticks celery, chopped

Mix all the warm ingredients with the seasoning. When cool, add the red pepper and celery. This salad can be served as a meal-in-one with some fresh avocado halves and a glass of carrot juice.

MARK'S RICE SALAD

2 cups cooked brown rice
½ cup black olives, pits removed
2–3 avocados, cubed
1 can navy or other beans (optional)
½ cup puréed tomato or chopped fresh tomato
1 red pepper, thinly sliced
1 cup lettuce, shredded
1–2 sticks celery, chopped

Combine all ingredients, adding the lettuce and avocado last to avoid a mushy salad.

I find that the salad is best if the rice has not been refrigerated but has been allowed to cool down to room temperature.

AVOCADO NOODLE SALAD

1 pound spiral noodles, cooked and drained

Combine with:

Mary-Ann's Organic Herb Salt or other herbal salt
and freshly ground black pepper
1 teaspoon oregano
4 tomatoes, diced
4 avocados, diced
Extra-virgin olive oil
Olives (optional)

Cook the noodles as directed on the packet. Steam the mushrooms lightly. Drain the noodles and add the oil, seasoning, and mushrooms. Either add the avocado, olives, and tomatoes immediately and serve as a hot dish, or allow the noodles to cool before adding the rest of the ingredients and serve as a salad.

WHOLE WHEAT PIZZA

(Makes 2 large round pizzas, or 1 very large square)
1 packet instant dry yeast (10 g or 0.35 oz)
1 cup whole wheat or brown flour
½ cup white bread flour
4 tablespoons extra-virgin olive oil
1 teaspoon sea salt
1 cup warm water

Place all ingredients in a food processor and mix using the plastic dough blade. Mix thoroughly until a ball of very pliable dough is formed. Add extra flour or water if the consistency is not quite right. Roll out into 2 large rounds and place on a baking sheet.

Blend 2 to 3 fresh ripe tomatoes with oregano, salt, and freshly ground black pepper in the food processor. Spread this over the pizza bases and bake at the highest oven temperature for 5 or 10 minutes. Remove and add the chopped vegetables of your choice, such as red pepper, olives, mushrooms, asparagus, artichokes, and zucchini. Return to the oven for about 10 minutes, cut into slices, and serve with a large fresh salad. Add sliced avocado after cooking and you will be amazed at how little you miss the cheese!

NEVER-FAIL WHOLE WHEAT BREAD

12 cups whole wheat flour
2 packets instant dry yeast (20 g or 0.7 oz)
3 teaspoons salt
3 teaspoons raw honey
6–7 cups of warm water (not hot)

Mix the flour, yeast, and salt in a large bowl. Dissolve the honey in a cup of water and add it to the dry ingredients. Keep adding the rest of the water until you have a sticky dough—do not knead. Divide the dough into 2 or 3 balls and place in greased bread pans (2 large or 3 medium pans). Cover with a cloth and allow to rise in a warm place for about 20 minutes. Bake at 392°F for 40 minutes.

Serve with a large salad. Remember to chew slowly so that the starch-digesting enzyme in your saliva can act upon the bread.

Special note: fresh oregano, mixed herbs, olives with pits removed, and grated zucchini can be added to the dough. Use each herb on its own or all of them together for a really different treat.

SPINACH LASAGNA

1 box flat lasagna sheets (egg-free)
1 cup ricotta cheese (about 250 g)
2 bunches spinach
½ bunch celery
5 tomatoes

Mary-Ann's Organic Seasoning Salt or Herb Salt
with freshly ground black pepper and a pinch of nutmeg
2 teaspoons oregano

Prepare the lasagna sheets according to the instructions on the packet. Steam the spinach lightly and chop finely. Add the ricotta cheese; mix with the spinach and season with salt, pepper, and nutmeg. Gently stir-fry the celery and tomatoes. Season with salt, pepper, and oregano, then layer in an ovenproof dish: first the spinach mixture, then the noodles, and then the tomato mixture. Add a sprinkling of Parmesan cheese and bake at 320°F–356°F (medium heat) for about 30 minutes.

This dish can be prepared in advance and can either be kept for a day in the fridge before baking, or it can be frozen.

Special note: you will notice that noodles and ricotta cheese are used in this recipe. Ricotta is very low in protein, as far as animal proteins go, and of all the cheeses it combines best with starch. This dish came about as a result of our love of lasagna. We hated the thought of never eating it again because of the meat and pasta combination. We now find this dish far more appealing than our old favorite. Remember that the seasoning and ingredients can be adjusted to suit your own taste.

QUICK SPAGHETTI AND TOMATO SAUCE

1 pound spaghetti noodles (egg-less)
1 can black olives, stoned and chopped (optional)
1–2 cans tomato purée (additive-free) or 6–8 fresh tomatoes,
finely chopped
½ cup carrots and celery, finely chopped (best in a food processor)
Oregano and basil, to taste

Cook spaghetti according to the instructions on the packet and drain well. For the sauce, cook the carrots and celery for 5 minutes and add the rest of the ingredients; heat through. If you like, a carton of organic fresh cream may be added at this stage but remember that it is high in animal fat. Season and serve on the spaghetti noodles.

Special note: this dish is a good alternative to Spaghetti Bolognese. Bear in mind that cooked tomatoes do become acidic during the cooking process but you counteract that with the carrots, celery, and the salad served with this meal.

FRESH TOMATO AND OLIVE PASTA

1 pound ripe tomatoes
1 bunch spring onions, chopped
½ cup black or green olives, pits removed and chopped
1 tablespoon capers
2 tablespoons parsley, chopped
1 teaspoon oregano
Mary-Ann's Organic Garlic & Herb Salt or 2 cloves garlic, crushed (optional)
½ cup extra-virgin olive oil

Chop the tomatoes and combine with all the other ingredients. This mixture can be heated gently or left to stand overnight and served as a cold sauce over your favorite freshly cooked pasta the next day. The second option is to serve the sauce raw as it is.

VEGETABLE AND HERB PASTA

1 cup zucchini, sliced into thin strips
1 cup broccoli, broken into small sprigs
1 cup green beans, sliced
2 tablespoons each of parsley, basil, and chives (or spring onions), chopped
1 pound pasta, cooked
Mary-Ann's Organic Herb Salt or other herbal salt

Steam the vegetables lightly. Mix together with the pasta, drizzle with olive oil, and serve.

ARTICHOKE AND OLIVE PASTA

1 pound noodles (egg-free)
4 large ripe tomatoes, chopped
1 can artichokes or asparagus
1 cup black olives in brine, pits removed and chopped
½ cup cold-pressed olive oil
½ cup fresh basil, chopped

Cook noodles according to the instructions on the packet and drain well. Drain the artichokes and mix with the other ingredients; serve either hot or cold with a fresh salad.

Step 5: Try to Eat Animal Protein No More Than Once a Day, Preferably No More Than Three Times a Week

PROTEIN DISHES

Protein dishes should be served with a fresh salad and any neutral vegetables. They should never accompany starch dishes. I have included very few recipes in this section for a good reason—all animal protein should be cooked as simply as possible, preferably grilled or roasted without added fat. Most people tend to be far too elaborate in their preparation of proteins—remember that simplest is best.

GRILLED FISH

Fish fillets, plain and not battered
Fresh lemon juice
Salt and pepper

Place the fish on a baking tray. Squeeze some lemon juice over each fillet and season with salt and pepper. Dot with butter and grill on the highest rack of the oven for 5 to 15 minutes, depending on the thickness of the fish. Serve with a fresh salad and any neutral vegetables. An avocado dip is an excellent sauce for grilled fish.

SAVORY BAKED FISH

Deep sea fish, such as hake fillets
1 tomato per person
1 bunch spring onions (enough for 4 people)
Fresh lemon juice
Herbal salt and black pepper

Set the oven at (medium to hot) 356°F. Place the fish fillets in an ovenproof dish. Layer the tomato, onions, and seasoning over the fish, and squeeze over some lemon juice. Bake for 20 to 30 minutes. Serve with salad and vegetables.

SOMETHING SWEET

Although sweets and desserts are not ideal from a food-combining point of view, the following "cheats" are suitable for special occasions—best eaten as an occasional snack or after a starch meal.

OAT SLICES

2 cups oats
2 cups whole wheat flour
2 cups coconut
1½ cups raw honey
1 teaspoon baking soda (bicarbonate of soda)
½ pound butter

Melt the butter and honey in a large pot on the stove. Mix the dry ingredients together and add them to the butter mixture. Press the mixture into a Swiss roll pan and bake for 20 to 25 minutes in a slow oven (284°F–320°F). Remove from the oven when done and cut into squares while still hot. Allow to cool in the pan.

Special note: these slices are better than most cookies as they contain a higher level of nutrients and fiber, but they should be regarded as treats and not everyday snacks. They do contain gluten.

WHEAT-FREE OAT SLICES

6 cups oats
2 cups rice or millet flour
½–1 cup coconut
½–1 cup sesame seeds
2 cups raw honey
1 pound butter

Melt the butter and mix with the honey. Add the dry ingredients and mix well. Press the mixture into a Swiss roll pan and bake at 356°F for 15 to 20 minutes.

Special note: remember that having a cupboard full of "goodies" is not the sign of a good mother. It is better to show your love for your family by not allowing them to eat badly. Cookies such as these should be occasional "treats."

DATE & COCONUT BALLS

2 cups dates
2–4 cups medium coconut, shredded

Soften the dates in a double boiler (place a heat-resistant dish inside a pot with water and bring the water to a boil).

When dates are soft, mash well, adding the coconut, mix by hand, and roll into balls. I keep these in the freezer as we find it makes them very "chewy." I often eat a few of these each day because they are so delicious.

Optional: add oats for a change if you are not gluten intolerant.

CAROB CAKE

5 tablespoons carob powder
1 cup water (or cream and water mixed)
5 organic egg yolks (the yolk digests better than the white does with starches, as it is low in protein)
½ pound butter
1 cup raw honey
1 teaspoon vanilla essence
1 cup whole wheat flour, sifted

2 teaspoons baking powder
½ teaspoon baking soda

Mix half the water, the carob powder, and 1 egg yolk together in a small pot and heat until just below boiling-point. Place the butter, honey, and remaining 4 egg yolks in a food processor and blend well. Add the carob mixture and the vanilla essence to the blender. Add the flour, baking powder, and baking soda and mix well (use the pulse facility on the blender to avoid over-processing). Add the rest of the water, alternating it with the flour. Pour the mixture into 2 standard greased round pans, and bake in a medium oven at 356°F for 25 to 30 minutes. Top with melted carob and whipped organic cream or mashed dates with cashew cream.

Special note: although cakes are not ideal, there will probably be the odd occasion where you will have to serve one. Egg yolks are used in this recipe as they are not as high in protein as egg whites, and they digest comfortably with starches.

CARROT CAKE

1 cup raw honey
1 cup cold-pressed extra-virgin vegetable oil
(a sweeter olive or sunflower oil works well)
3 eggs
1½ cups whole wheat flour
2 teaspoons baking powder
2 teaspoons cinnamon
1 teaspoon baking soda
1 cup mashed bananas
1 cup carrots, finely grated
½ cup pecans

Cream honey, oil, and eggs; sift the flour, cinnamon, and soda together. Add the sugar mixture and the rest of the ingredients to the flour mixture. Mix well. Bake in 2 round cake tins for about 25 minutes at 356°F.

Special note: although not a wonderful combination, this is a better alternative than "normal" cake as it is very nutritious.

HOMEMADE ICE CREAM

1 liter organic fresh cream
1 can (about 2 cups) coconut cream or milk
(buy one that has no preservatives)
1 cup raw honey
1 teaspoon natural vanilla essence

Blend with a whisk and pour either into an ice cream machine or a freezer dish. Remove when frozen and blend in a food processor until smooth and re-freeze. Do this twice more and serve.

CHRISTMAS ICE CREAM (TO BE EATEN ANY TIME OF THE YEAR)

2 cups organic fresh cream or soymilk
½–1 cup raw honey
½ cup almonds
2–3 bananas
1 teaspoon cinnamon
½ cup raisins
½ cup sultanas
½ cup dried peaches, chopped

Set the cream aside and blend the remaining ingredients in a food processor until fairly fine textured (it depends on how many bits and pieces you want in your ice cream). Add the cream and blend quickly until well-mixed. Freeze as you would ordinary ice cream. Instead of the cream, you could use soy milk or a mixture of cream and soy milk, or even cream, soy milk, and filtered water.

ALCOHOL-FREE SANGRIA

2 pints unsweetened, unpreserved grape juice
1 cup prune juice (Make by soaking ½ pound prunes
in 4 cups filtered water for at least 24 hours, longer if thicker syrup
required. Drain and use the syrup. Eat the prunes as a separate meal
with sweet fruit.)
1 teaspoon cinnamon
½ teaspoon ginger

¼ *teaspoon nutmeg*

Rind of 1 lemon and 1 orange—use a zester or just cut into
very thin strips (You can also add the juice of the lemon
and orange if you like.)

Combine with crushed ice and dilute with sparkling mineral water
as required.

Or:

Leave out the ice and sparkling water and heat through and
serve hot in winter as a mulled "wine."

(Most people are convinced these two options contain alcohol.)

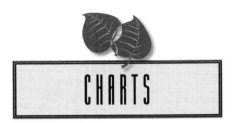

CHARTS

Nuts and Vegetables — Nutritive Value Chart 1

Food	Grams	Water %	Food Energy (Calories) Kj	Protein g	Fat g	Saturated g
NUTS (shelled)						
Almonds (1 cup)	130	4.7	3254	24.18	70.46	5.58
Brazil Nuts (1 cup)	120	4.6	3286	17.16	80.28	20.50
Cashews (1 cup)	140	5.2	3287	24.08	63.98	10.71
Coconut, shredded (½ cup)	40	3.5	1108	2.88	25.96	22.46
Hazelnuts (1 cup)	115	5.8	3052	14.49	71.76	5.13
Pecans (1 cup)	120	3.4	3451	11.04	85.44	6.95
Sunflower Seeds (½ cup)	80	4.8	1875	19.2	37.84	4.77
Walnuts (1 cup)	120	3.5	3270	11.84	76.8	8.35

VEGETABLES (½ cup)

String Beans (C)	120	92.4	126	1.92	0.24	0.06
Broccoli (C)	75	91.3	82	2.33	0.23	-
Cabbage (C)	80	93.9	67	0.88	0.16	-
Cabbage (R)	80	92.4	80	1.04	0.16	-
Carrots (C)	80	91.2	104	0.72	0.16	-
Carrots (R)	80	88.2	141	0.88	0.16	-
Cauliflower (C)	80	92.8	74	1.84	0.16	-
Cauliflower (R)	80	91	90	2.16	0.16	-
Cucumber	50	95.7	30	0.3	0.05	-
Green Peas	85	81.5	252	4.59	0.34	0.16
Lettuce	100	95.9	53	1.0	0.2	0.03
Potato (Boiled)	90	82.8	245	1.71	0.09	0.02
Summer Gem Squash	75	95.5	44	0.68	0.08	-
Winter Hubbard Squash	125	88.8	199	1.38	0.38	-
Spinach	90	92	86	2.70	0.27	0.04
Sweet Potato	145	72	526	1.60	0.87	0.42
Tomato	200	93.5	184	2.2	0.4	-

Nuts and Vegetables — Nutritive Value Chart 2

	Grams	Monounsat g	Polyunsat g	Carbohydrates g	Calcium mg	Iron mg	Vitamin A iu
NUTS (shelled)							
Almonds (1 cup)	130	48.22	13.21	6.8	304	6.11	0
Brazil Nuts (1 cup)	120	26.33	29.93	5.16	223	4.08	0
Cashews (1 cup)	140	42.83	4.02	39.1	53	5.32	140
Coconut Desic. (125 ml)	40	1.50	0.47	2.5	10	1.32	0
Hazelnuts (1 cup)	115	55.6	7.48	7.9	240	3.91	0
Pecans (250 ml)	120	49.33	20.42	17.5	88	2.88	156
Sunflower Seeds (125 ml)	80	7.0	24.26	12.7	96	5.68	40
Walnuts (1 cup)	120	11.96	52.42	11.0	119	3.72	36
VEGETABLES							
Green Beans (C)	120	0.01	0.17	3.1	60	0.72	648
Broccoli (C) (1 cup)	75	-	-	0.8	66	0.6	1.875

Cabbage (C) (1 cup)	80	-	-	1.2	35	0.24	104
Cabbage (R) (1 cup)	80	-	-	3.2	3269	0.32	104
Carrots (C) (½ cup)	80	-	-	5.0	30	0.56	8.800
Cauliflower (C) (½ cup)	80	-	-	1.4	17	0.56	48
Cauliflower (R) (½ cup)	80	-	-	2.1	20	0.88	48
Cucumber (5 slices)	50	-	-	1.4	9	0.15	0
Green Peas (C)	85	0.14	0.04	6.0	20	1.53	459
Lettuce	100	0.01	0.10	0.6	19	0.5	330
Potato (Boiled)	90	0.01	0.06	12.2	5	0.45	0
Summer Squash (C)	75	-	-	2.0	19	0.3	293
Winter Squash (C)	125	-	-	10.1	25	0.63	4.375
Spinach (C)	90	0.03	0.21	0.2	84	1.98	7.290
Sweet Potato (C)	145	0.07	0.36	29.1	30	0.87	9.667
Tomato	200	-	-	6.4	26	1.0	1.800

R = raw C = cooked   - = No reliable data

Nuts and Vegetables — Nutritive Value Chart 3

	Grams	Thiamin mg	Riboflavin mg	Nicotinic Acid mg	Vitamin B6 mg	Folic Acid mg	Ascorbic Acid (Vitamin C) (mg)
NUTS (shelled) — Nuts–1 cup; Seeds & Coconut–½ cup							
Almonds	130	0.31	1.20	4.55	0.13	125	tr
Brazil Nuts	120	1.15	0.14	1.92	0.212	5	tr
Cashews	140	0.60	0.35	2.52	-	95	0
Coconut Desic.	40	0.02	0.02	0.24	0.018	10	0
Hazelnuts	115	0.53	-	1.04	1.012	132	tr
Pecans	120	1.03	0.16	1.08	0.22	29	2
Sunflower Seeds	80	1.56	0.18	4.32	1.0	186	0
Walnuts	120	0.40	0.16	1.08	1.104	100	2
VEGETABLES							
Green Beans (C)	120	0.08	0.11	0.6	0.068	59	14
Broccoli (C)	75	0.07	0.15	0.6	0.084	71	68
Cabbage (C)	80	0.03	0.03	0.24	0.08	28	26
Cabbage (R)	80	0.04	0.04	0.24	0.08	46	38
Carrots (C)	80	0.04	0.04	0.40	0.072	6	5
Carrots (R)	80	0.05	0.04	0.48	0.14	14	6
Cauliflower (C)	80	0.07	0.06	0.48	0.126	51	44
Cauliflower (R)	80	0.09	0.08	0.56	0.197	38	62

Cucumber (5 slices)	50	0.02	0.02	0.1	0.024	10	6
Green Peas (C)	85	0.24	0.09	1.96	0.078	45	17
Lettuce	100	0.05	0.03	0.2	0.04	56	4
Potato (Boiled)	90	0.07	0.03	0.99	0.131	9	13
Summer Squash (C)	75	0.04	0.06	0.6	0.038	8	8
Winter Squash (C)	125	0.05	0.13	0.50	0.159	34	10
Spinach (C)	90	0.06	0.13	0.45	0.087	68	25
Sweet Potato (C)	145	0.12	0.06	0.87	0.189	36	22
Tomato	200	0.12	0.08	1.4	0.220	56	46

R = raw   C = cooked   tr = Trace or small amount   - =No reliable data

Fruit — Nutritive Value Chart 1

	Apples	Apricots	Avocados	Bananas	Cherries	Dates	Dried Figs	Goose-berries	Passion Fruit
Grams (g)	160	50	125	80	68	50	20	75	60
Water (%)	83.9	86.4	74.3	74.3	80.8	22.5	28.4	87.9	72.9
Food Energy (Calories) (Kj)	392	101	843	307	204	576	214	140	245
Protein (g)	0.32	0.70	2.5	0.8	0.82	1.0	0.62	0.68	1.32
Fat (g)	0.64	0.2	19.13	0.40	0.68	0.25	0.24	0.45	0.42
Saturated (g)	0.10	0.02	3.05	0.15	0.15	-	0.05	0.03	-
Monounsat (g)	0.03	0.09	12.01	0.03	0.18	-	0.05	0.04	-
Polyunsat (g)	0.18	0.04	2.45	0.07	0.20	-	0.11	0.24	-
Carbohydrate (g)	19.5	4.5	6.6	16.3	10.3	32.8	9.9	5.7	4.5
Calcium (mg)	11.0	7.0	14.0	5.0	10.0	16.0	29.0	19.0	7.0
Iron (mg)	0.32	0.25	1.25	0.24	0.27	0.6	0.44	0.23	0.96
Vitamin A (iu)	85.0	1306	765.0	65.0	146.0	25.0	27.0	218.0	420.0
Thiamin (mg)	0.03	0.02	0.14	0.04	0.03	0.05	0.01	0.03	tr
Riboflavin (mg) 0,02	0.02	0.15	0.08	0.04	0.05	0.01	0.02	0.08	-
Nicotinic Acid (mg)	0.16	0.03	2.38	0.4	0.27	1.1	0.14	0.23	0.9
Vitamin B6 (mg)	0.077	0.027	0.35	0.462	0.024	0.096	0.045	0.06	-
Folic Acid (mg)	5.0	5.0	78.0	15.0	3.0	7.0	2.0	-	-
Ascorbic Acid (mg) (Vitamin C)	10.0	5.0	10.0	7.0	5.0	-	tr	21.0	18.0

tr = Trace or small amount   - =No reliable data

Fruit — Nutritive Value Chart 2

	Grapefruit	Grapes	Guavas	Kiwi	Lemons	Loquats	Litchis (Yellow)	Mangoes	Melons
Grams (g)	120	250	75	100	75	60	80	350	250
Water (%)	90.9	80.6	86.1	80.5	89.0	86.7	81.8	81.7	89.8
Food Energy (Calories) (Kj)	161	743	158	281	92	118	221	956	370
Protein (g)	0.72	1.75	0.60	1.0	0.83	0.24	0.64	1.75	2.25
Fat (g)	0.12	1.5	0.45	0.6	0.23	0.12	0.32	1.05	0.75
Saturated (g)	0.01	0.05	0.13	-	0.03	0.02	-	0.25	-
Monounsat (g)	0.01	0.05	0.05	-	0.01	0.01	-	0.35	-
Polyunsat (g)	0.02	0.43	0.19	-	0.08	0.05	-	0.18	-
Carbohydrate (g)	9.0	40.3	4.7	14.2	6.8	7.0	12.8	53.9	17.0
Calcium (mg)	14.0	28.0	15.0	29.0	20.0	10.0	4.0	35.0	28.0
Iron (mg)	0.12	0.75	0.23	0.4	0.45	0.18	0.24	0.35	0.5
Vitamin A (iu)	149.0	183.0	593.0	-	22.0	917.0	0	13629	8060
Thiamin (mg)	0.05	0.23	0.04	0.02	0.03	0.01	0.01	0.21	0.1
Riboflavin (mg)	0.02	0.15	0.04	0.01	0.02	0.01	0.06	0.21	0.05
Nicotinic Acid (mg)	0.36	0.75	0.9	0.2	0.08	0.12	0.48	2.1	1.5
Vitamin B6 (mg)	0.05	0.275	0.107	-	0.06	-	-	0.469	0.288
Folic Acid (mg)	12.0	10.0	-	-	8.0	-	-	-	43.0
Ascorbic Acid (mg) (Vitamin C)	41.0	28.0	138.0	118.0	40.0	1.0	58.0	98.0	108.0

- = No reliable data

Fruit — Nutritive Value Chart 3

	Melons (Green)	Tangerines	Oranges	Papaya	Peaches	Pears	Pineapples	Plums	Prickly Pears
Grams (g)	250	105	130	80	150	220	85	50	75
Water (%)	89.7	87.6	86.8	88.8	87.7	83.8	86.5	85.2	87.6
Food Energy (Calories) (Kj)	370	193	256	129	270	543	176	115	129
Protein (g)	1.25	0.63	1.17	0.48	1.05	0.88	0.34	0.4	0.53
Fat (g)	0.25	0.21	0.13	0.08	0.15	0.88	0.34	0.30	0.45
Saturated (g)	-	0.02	0.03	0.03	0.02	0.04	0.03	0.03	-
Monounsat (g)	-	0.03	0.03	0.03	0.05	0.18	0.04	0.21	-
Polyunsat (g)	-	0.04	0.04	0.02	0.08	0.20	0.13	0.07	-
Carbohydrate (g)	19.0	9.8	12.7	7.1	14.9	27.7	9.3	5.5	5.9
Calcium (mg)	15.0	15.0	52.0	19.0	8.0	24.0	6.0	2.0	42.0
Iron (mg)	0.25	0.11	0.13	0.08	0.15	0.66	0.34	0.05	0.23
Vitamin A (iu)	100.0	966.0	267.0	1611	803.0	44.0	20.0	161.0	38.0
Thiamin (mg)	0.2	0.12	0.12	0.02	0.03	0.04	0.08	0.02	0.01
Riboflavin (mg)	0.05	0.02	0.05	0.02	0.06	0.09	0.03	0.05	0.05
Nicotinic Acid (mg)	1.5	0.21	0.39	0.24	1.5	0.22	0.34	0.25	0.38
Vitamin B6 (mg)	0.148	0.07	0.078	0.015	0.027	0.04	0.074	0.041	-
Folic Acid (mg)	133.0	21.0	39.0	-	5.0	15.0	9.0	1.0	-
AscorbicAcid (Vitamin C) (mg)	63.0	33.0	69.0	50.0	11.0	9.0	13.0	5.0	11.0

Food-Combining Chart

PROTEINS, NEUTRAL VEGETABLES, & STARCH

Guidelines When Eating Protein, Neutral Vegetables, & Starch:

- *Protein-starch* combinations are difficult to digest and are prone to fermentation
- Eat one *protein* meal at a time (preferably once a day only) as a main course with a large salad and/or neutral vegetable
- Eat one *starch* at a time as a meal with a large salad and/or neutral vegetables
- *Fats* (butter, cream, cold-pressed oils) should be eaten in small quantities and can be combined with protein, neutral vegetables, and starch
- Wait at least *3 hours* after eating the foods below before eating *fruit* again
- All *legumes* (dried beans, garbonzo beans, lentils, peanuts, etc.) are high in both starch and protein and are therefore prone to fermentation, resulting in digestive discomfort

Don't Mix Well Together

Good Combination   Good Combination

Proteins	Neutral Vegetables	Starch
#Dairy Products	Artichoke, Asparagus, Avocado	Barley
#Eggs	Beetroot, Broccoli	Bread
#Fish	Brussels Sprouts	Buckwheat
*Meat	Cabbage, Cucumber	Cereals
*Milk	Eggplant	Jerusalem Artichoke
Nuts (Incl. Coconut)	Fennel, Garlic	Maize/Corn
#Poultry	Squash (Including Gem & Butternut)	Millet
Seeds	Green Beans	Oats
Unprocessed Cheese	Herbs, Leeks, Lettuce	Pasta
#Yogurt	Mushrooms, Okra	Potatoes
	Peas (Fresh)	Rice
	Peppers (Green, Yellow, & Red)	Rice cakes
	Pumpkin, Radishes	Rye
	Shallots, Spinach, Spring Onions	Sweet Potatoes
	Sprouts, Tomatoes, Turnips	Wheat
	Watercress	
	Zucchini	

\# = Minimize consumption
* = Once or twice per week in small quantities

Food-Combining Chart

FRUITS

Guidelines When Eating Fruit:

- Your daily menu should consist of 75% raw fruits and vegetables
- Fruit can replace any meal
- Eat fruit by itself on an empty stomach
- Wait 40–60 minutes after eating fruit before eating any other food
- Nuts can be eaten with any acid fruit
- Fruit can be eaten 3–4 hours after any other food
- All melons (yellow melon, green melon, watermelon) are best eaten alone

Don't Mix Well Together

Good
Combination

Good
Combination

Acid Fruit	Sub-Acid Fruit	Sweet Fruit
Gooseberries	Apples	Bananas
Grapefruit	Apricots	Dates
Guavas	Berries	Dried Fruit
Kiwi	Cherries	Figs
Kumquats	Grapes	Papaya
Lemons	Litchis	Papino
Limes	Loquats	Persimmons
Melons	Mongoes	Prunes
Oranges	Nectarines	Raisins
Pineapples	Peaches	Seedless Grapes
Passion Fruit	Pears	Sultanas (Unbleached)
Pomegranates	Plums	
Quinces	Prickly Pears	
Strawberries		
Tangerines		
Watermelon		

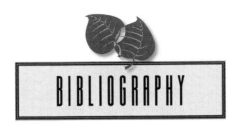

BIBLIOGRAPHY

Abercrombie, M. *Dictionary of Biology*. U.S.: Penguin Books, 1980.

Airola, Dr. Paavo. *How to Keep Slim, Healthy, and Young with Juice Fasting*. U.S.: Health Plus, 1990.

April, E. W. *Anatomy*. 2nd ed. U.S.: Williams and Wilkins, 1990.

Astor, Stephen. *Hidden Food Allergies*. U.S.: Avery Publishing Group, 1988.

Bailey, Covert. *The New Fit or Fat*. Boston: Houghton Mifflin Company, 1991.

Balch, J. F. *Prescription for Nutritional Healing*. U.S.: Avery Publishing Group, 1990.

Ballentine, R. *Diet and Nutrition: A Holistic Approach*. U.S.: The Himalayan International Institute, 1989.

Banik, Allen B. *Your Water and Your Health*. U.S.: Keats Publishing, 1990.

Barbor, T. *Alcohol*. U.S.: Burke Publishing Co., 1988.

Barilla, Jean. *The Nutrition Superbook*. Vol. 1. U.S.: Keats Publishing, 1995.

Berkow, R. *The Merck Manual of Medical Information*. U.S.: Pocket Books, 1999.

Bethel, May. *The Healing Power of Natural Foods*. U.S.: Wilshire Book Co., 1978.

Bieler, Henry G. *Food Is Your Best Medicine*. U.S.: Random House, 1983.

Bircher-Benner, Dr. M. *The Prevention of Incurable Disease*. U.S.: Keats Publishing, 1978.

Bragg, Paul C. *Healthful Eating without Confusion*. U.S.: Health Science.

Bragg, Paul C. *Nature's Way to Health*. U.S.: Health Science.

Bragg, Paul C. *The Miracle of Fasting*. U.S.: Health Science.

Bragg, Paul C. *The Shocking Truth About Water*. U.S.: Health Science.

Braly, Dr. James. *Food Allergy and Nutrition*. Connecticut: Keats Publishing, 1992.

Brand, Dr. Paul. *Fearfully and Wonderfully Made*. U.S.: Zondervan Publishing House, 1984.

Brandt, Johanna. *The Fasting Book*. South Africa: De Nationale Pers, 1921.

Brandt, Johanna. *The Grape Cure*. U.S.: Ehret Literature Publishing Co., 1983.

Braverman, Eric R. *The Healing Nutrients Within*. U.S.: Keats Publishing, 1987.

Bricklin, M. *Prevention's Practical Encyclopedia of Walking for Health*. U.S.: Rodale Press, 1992.

Brighthope, Ian. *The AIDS Fighters*. U.S.: Keats Publishing, 1988.

Brown, G. I. *Introduction to Organic Chemistry*. U.K.: Longman, 1977.

Brown, Harold R. *Fast Way to Health and Vigour*. South Africa: Healthy Life Publishers, 1973.

Budd, Martin L. *Low Blood Sugar*. U.K.: Thorsons, 1984.

Budd, Martin. *Diets to Help Diabetes*. U.K.: Thorsons, 1994.

Bueno, Lee. *Fast Your Way to Health*. U.S.: Whitaker House, 1982.

Buist, Robert. *Food Chemical Sensitivity*. U.S.: Harper and Row, 1988.

Button, John. *How to Be Green*. U.K.: Century, 1989.

Campbell, T. Colin. *The China Study*. Dallas: BenBella Books, 2005.

Carper, Jean. *The Food Pharmacy*. U.K.: Simon and Schuster Ltd., 1988.

Carrol, Dr. S. *Complete Family Guide to Healthy Living*. U.K.: Dorling Kindersley, 1992.

Chadwick, T. F. *Chemistry*. U.K.: George Allen and Unwin, 1974.

Chaitow, Leon. *Thorsons Guide to Amino Acids*. U.K.: Thorsons, 1991.

Cheraskin, E. *Diet and Disease*. U.S.: Keats Publishing, 1968.

Cheraskin, Emanuel. *The Vitamin Controversy: Questions and Answers*. U.S.: Bio-Communications Press, 1988.

Chetley, Andrew. *A Healthy Business*. U.K.: Zed Books Ltd., 1990.

Clark, Hulda Regehr. *The Cure for All Cancers*. U.S.: New Century Press, 1993.

Clark, Linda. *Stay Younger Longer*. U.S.: Pyramid Books, 1971.

Clobert, John. *Walking in Divine Health*. U.S.: Creation House, 1996.

Colgan, Dr. Michael. *Your Personal Vitamin Profile*. U.K.: Blond & Briggs, 1983.

Collings, Jillie. *The Ordinary Person's Guide to Extraordinary Health*. U.K.: Aurum Press, 1997.

Contreras, Francisco. *Health in the 21st Century*. U.S.: Interpacific Press, 1997.

Contreras, Francisco. *The Hope of Living Cancer FREE*. U.S.: Siloam Press, 1999.

Cotton, F. A. *Basic Inorganic Chemistry*. Canada: John Wiley and Sons, 1987.

Cox, Peter. *The New Why You Don't Need to Eat Meat*. London: Bloomsbury, 1992.

Dufty, William. *Sugar Blues*. New York: Warner Books, 1993.

Dunne, L. J. *Nutrition Almanac*. 3rd ed. R. R. Donnelley and Sons Company, 1990.

Erasmus, Udo. *Fats that Heal, Fats that Kill*. Canada: Alive Books, 1993.

Fielder, John L. *Milk: A Danger to Your Health*. (Booklet)

Forbes, Alec. *The Famous Bristol Detox Diet for Cancer Patients*. U.S.: Keats Publishing, 1984.

Ford, Norman D. *18 Natural Ways to Lower Cholesterol in 30 Days*. U.S.: Keats Publishing, 1992.

Fredericks, Carlton. *New Low Blood Sugar and You*. New York: Perigee Books, 1985.

Fuhrman, Dr. Joel. *Fasting and Eating for Health*. New York: St. Martin's Press, 1995.

Garrett, L. *The Coming Plague*. U.S.: Penguin Books, 1995.

Garrison, R. H. *The Nutrition Desk Reference*. 2nd ed. U.S.: Keats Publishing, 1990.

Gilbert, R. *Caffeine*. U.S.: Burke Publishing Co., 1988.

Goodman, Sandra. *Vitamin C: The Master Nutrient*. U.S.: Keats Publishing, 1991.

Graham, D. N. *Nutrition and Athletic Performance*. U.S. 1999.

Granger, Laura. *Nutrition for Teeth and Bones*. U.K.: Foulsham, 1992.

Grant, Belinda. *Alternative Health: The A-Z of Natural Healthcare*. U.K.: Optima Books, 1993.

Grant, Doris. *Food Combining for Health*. U.K.: Thorsons, 1985.

Gray, H. *Gray's Anatomy*. U.S.: Running Press, 1974.

Greer, Rita. *Diets to Help Gluten and Wheat Allergy*. U.K.: Thorsons, 1993.

Guyton, Arthur C. *Textbook of Medical Physiology*. U.S.: Saunders College Publishing, 1986.

Haas, Dr. R. *Eat to Win*. U.K.: Penguin, 1987.

Hagiwara, Dr. Yoshihide. *Green Barley Essence*. Connecticut: Keats Publishing, 1985.

Hawkins, M. *Rebounding for Health and Fitness*. U.K.: Thorsons, 1993.

Hay, Dr. William Howard. *Weight Control*. London: George G. Harrap & Co., 1936.

Hirschmann, Jane R. *Overcoming Overeating*. London: Mandarin, 1990.

Hoffer, A. *Orthomolecular Medicine for Physicians*. U.S.: Keats Publishing, 1989.

Holford, Patrick. *Optimum Nutrition Workbook*. U.K.: ION Press, 1992.

Holford, Patrick. *The H Factor*. U.K.: Piatkus, 2003.

Holford, Patrick. *The Whole Health Manual*. U.K.: Thorsons, 1988.

Horne, Ross. *Health and Survival in the 21st Century*. Australia: Happy Landings, 1992.

Horne, Ross. *The Health Revolution*. 4th ed. Australia: Happy Landings, 1985.

Jensen, B. *The Chemistry of Man*. U.S.: Bernard Jensen Publishers, 1983.

Jensen, Dr. Bernard. *Arthritis, Rheumatism, and Osteoporosis*. U.S.: Bernard Jensen Enterprises, 1986.

Jensen, Dr. Bernard. *Foods That Heal*. U.S.: Avery Publishing Group, 1993.

Junshi, C. T. *Diet, Lifestyle, and Mortality in China*. U.S.: People's Publishing House, 1990.

Katz, Denise. *The No Smoking Diet*. U.K.: Kyle Cathie Ltd., 1993.

Kenton, Lesley. *The X Factor Diet*. London: Vermilion, 2002.

Kenton, Susan. *Endless Energy*. U.K.: Vermillion, 1994.

Kordel, Lelord. *Eat Right and Live Longer, Look Younger, Be More Vital*. U.S.: Health Today Books, 1968.

Lanctot, G. *The Medical Mafia*. U.S.: Here's the Key, 1995.

Lappe, Frances Moore. *Diet for a Small Planet*. U.S.: Ballantine Books, 1991.

Lawrence, Marilyn. *Fed Up and Hungry*. London: The Women's Press, 1989.

Lee, John R. *What your Doctor May Not Tell You About Breast Cancer*. U.S.: Warner Books, 2003.

Lindner, Peter G. *Mind Over Platter*. U.S.: Wilshire Book Company, 1963.

Long, R. Y. *Homestudy Course in the New Nutrition*. U.S.: Keats Publishing, 1989.

Mackarness, Dr. Richard. *Not All in the Mind*. U.K.: Thorsons, 1994.

Malstrom, Stan D. *Own Your Own Body*. U.S.: Keats Publishing, 1980.

Marieb, E. N. *Human Anatomy and Physiology*. U.S.: The Benjamin/Cummings Publishing Company, 1989.

Mayes, Adrienne. *The A-Z of Nutritional Health*. U.K.: Thorsons, 1991.

Mayes, Kathleen. *The Complete Guide to Digestive Health*. U.K.: Thorsons, 1990.

McArdle, William D. *Exercise Physiology*. U.S.: Lea and Ferbiger, 1991.

McTaggart, Lynne. *What Doctors Don't Tell You*. U.S.: Avon Books, 1999.

Meek, Jennifer. *How to Boost your Immune System*. U.K.: ION Press, 1988.

Meek, Jennifer. *Immune Power*. U.K.: Macdonald and Co., 1990.

Mendelsohn, R. S. *Confessions of a Medical Heretic*. U.S.: Warner Books, 1980.

Meyer, B. J. *Fruit for Thought*. South Africa: HAUM Publishers, 1979.

Meyer, B. J. *Human Physiology*. South Africa: Creda Press, 1994.

Millstone, E. *Additives: A Guide for Everyone*. U.K.: Penguin Books, 1988.

Mindell, Earl. *The Vitamin Bible*. U.K.: Arlington Books, 1993.

Moore, J. W. *Chemistry*. U.S.: McGrawHill, 1978.

Morril, J. S. *Science, Physiology, and Nutrition for the Non-scientist*. U.S.: Orange Grove Pub., 2000.

Morter, Dr. M. Ted. *Your Health, Your Choice*. U.S.: Life Time Books, 1990.

Mumby, Dr. Keith. *Food Allergies and Environmental Illness*. U.K.: Thorsons, 1993.

Munro, Daniel C. *You Can Live Longer Than You Think*. U.S.: Bartholomew House, 1948.

Nelson, Dennis. *Food Combining Simplified*. Booklet, 1988.

Newbold, Dr. H. L. *Nutrition for Your Nerves*. U.S.: Keats Publishing, 1993.

Nicol, Rosemary. *Sleep Like a Dream*. U.K.: Sheldon Press, 1993.

Nostrand, Carol A. *Junk Food to Real Food*. U.S.: Keats Publishing, 1994.

Ornish, Dr. Dean. *Eat More, Weigh Less*. London: HarperCollins, 1993.

Ornish, Dr. Dean. *Dr. Dean Ornish's Program for Reversing Heart Disease*. U.S.: Ballantine Books, 1996.

Orr, M. H. *The Language of Science*. South Africa: Butterworths, 1994.

Page, Melvin E. *Your Body Is Your Best Doctor*. U.S.: Keats Pulishing, 1991.

Passwater, Richard A. *Cancer Prevention and Nutritional Therapies*. U.S.: Keats Publishing, 1993.

Payne, Dr. Mark. *Super Health*. U.K.: Thorsons, 1992.

Pfeiffer, Carl C. *Mental and Elemental Nutrients*. U.S.: Keats Publishing, 1975.

Pfeiffer, Dr. Carl C. *Total Nutrition: Eat Well and Stay Well*. U.K.: Granada, 1983.

Philpott, William H. *Brain Allergies*. U.S.: Keats Publishing, 1987.

Pottenger, Francis M. *Pottenger's Cats*. U.S.: Price-Pottenger Nutrition Foundation, 1983.

Price, W. A. *Nutrition and Physical Degeneration*. U.S.: Keats Publishing, 1989.

Readers Digest. *Eat Better, Live Better*. South Africa: Readers Digest, 1985.

Rifkin, Jeremy. *Beyond Beef*. U.K.: Thorsons, 1992.

Robbins, John. *The Food Revolution*. Berkeley, California: Conari Press, 2001.

Robbins, John. *Diet for a New America*. U.S.: Stillpoint Publishing, 1987.

Rosenveld, Lloyd. *Can A Gluten-Free Diet Help? How?* U.S.: Keats Publishing, 1992.

Rothera, Ellen. *Perhaps It's an Allergy*. U.K.: W. Foulsham & Co., 1988.

Saunders, W. B. *Dorland's Pocket Medical Dictionary*. 25th ed. U.S. 1995.

Saynor, Dr. Reg. *The Eskimo Diet*. U.K.: Ebury Press, 1990.

Scharffenberg, John A. *Problems with Meat*. U.S.: Woodbridge Press Publishing Company, 1982.

Schlosser, Eric. *Fast Food Nation*. London: Penguin Books, 2002.

Schroeder, Henry A. *The Poisons Around Us*. U.S.: Keats Publishing, 1978.

Seaman, Barbara. *The Doctors' Case Against the Pill*. California: Hunter House, 1995.

Serfontein, Dr. Willem. *Feel Better, Live Longer*. South Africa: Tafelberg Publishers, 2003.

Shackleton, Basil. *The Grape Cure: A Living Testament*. U.K.: Thorsons, 1983.

Sharma, Dr. Nandkishore. *Milk: A Silent Killer*. U.S.: Health Science Publications, 1992.

Shelton, Herbert M. *Natural Hygiene. The Pristine Way of Life*. U.S.: American Natural Hygiene Society, 1994.

Shelton, Herbert M. *The Original Natural Hygiene Weight Loss*. Connecticut: Keats Publishing, 1986.

Shelton, Herbert M. *Fasting Can Save your Life*. U.S.: Natural Hygiene Press, 1996.

Shelton, Herbert M. *Fasting for Renewal of Life*. U.S.: Natural Hygiene Press, 1995.

Shelton, Herbert M. *Health for the Millions*. U.S.: American Natural Hygiene Society, 1996.

Shelton, Herbert M. *Superior Nutrition*. U.S.: Willow Publishing, 1987.

Shelton, Herbert M. *The Science and Fine Art of Fasting*. U.S.: Natural Hygiene Press, 1993.

Shelton, Herbert M. *The Science and Fine Art of Food and Nutrition*. U.S.: Natural Hygiene Press, 1996.

Shelton, Herbert M. *The Science and Fine Art of Natural Hygiene*. U.S.: American Natural Hygiene Society, 1994.

Sinden, Dr. Andre. *Health Won*. South Africa: Abraham Kruger Hoogland, 1994.

Smith, Dr. M. *The New Dictionary of Symptoms*. U.K.: HarperCollins, 1993.

Smyth, Angela. *Seasonal Affective Disorder*. London: Unwin Books, 1990.

Solomon, Eldra. *Biology*. 3rd ed. U.S.: Saunders College Publishing, 1993.

Soltanoff, Jack. *Natural Healing*. U.S.: Warner Books, 1989.

Stewart, M. *Beat Sugar Craving*. London: Vermilion, 1992.

Swope, Dr. Mary Ruth. *Are You Sick & Tired of Feeling Sick & Tired?* U.S.: Whitaker House, 1984.

Swope, Dr. Mary Ruth. *Green Leaves of Barley*. U.S.: Swope Enterprises, 1990.

Swope, Dr. Mary Ruth. *The Roots and Fruits of Fasting*. U.S.: Swope Enterprises, 1998.

Taylor, Rene. *Hunza Health Secrets*. Connecticut: Keats Publishing, 1964.

Thomas, Pat. *Cleaning Yourself to Death*. U.K.: Newleaf, 2001.

Tobe, John H. *Margarine*. U.S.: Provoker Press, 1976.

Tortora, G. J. *Principles of Anatomy and Physiology*. U.S.: HarperCollins, 1993.

Trattler, Ross. *Better Health Through Natural Healing*. U.K.: Thorsons, 1987.

Travis, J.W. *Wellness Workbook*. 2nd ed. U.S.: Ten Speed Press, 1988.

Trickett, Shirley. *Coming off Tranquilizers & Sleeping Pills*. U.K.: Thorsons, 1991.

Trickett, Shirley. *Irritable Bowel Syndrome & Diverticulosis*. U.K.: Thorsons, 1990.

Trum Hunter, Beatrice. *Additives Book*. U.S.: Keats Publishing, 1982.

Turner, Roger Newman. *Diets to Help Asthma and Hay Fever*. U.K.: Thorsons, 1993.

Turner, Roger Newman. *Diets to Help Control Cholesterol*. U.K.: Thorsons, 1993.

Van Straten, Michael. *The Super Foods Diet Book*. U.K.: Dorling Kindersley, 1992.

Veith, Walter J. *Diet and Health*. Stuttgart: Medpharm, 1998.

Virkler, Mark and Patti. *Go Natural*. U.S.: Destiny Image Publishers, 1994.

Vogel, Dr. H. C. A. *The Nature Doctor*. U.S.: Keats Publishing, 1991.

Walker, N. W. *Water Can Undermine Your Health*. U.S.: Norwalk Press, 1974.

Walker, Norman W. *Natural Weight Control*. Arizona: Norwalk Press, 1981.

Webb, Tony. *Food Irradiation: The Facts*. U.K.: Thorsons, 1987.

Weil, Dr. Andrew. *Eating Well for Optimum Health*. Great Britain: Little Brown Books, 2000.

Weil, Dr. Andrew. *Ask Dr. Weil: Your Top Health Concerns*. U.S.: Ballantine Books, 1997.

Weitz, Martin. *A Guide to Ineffective and Hazardous Medical Treatment: Health Shock*. U.K.: David and Charles Publishers, 1980.

Werbach, M. R. *Nutritional Influences on Illness*. U.S.: Keats Publishers, 1988.

Whitfield, R. C. *A Guide to Understanding Basic Organic Reactions*. U.K.: Longman, 1972.

Wigmore, Ann. *Be Your Own Doctor*. U.S.: Avery Publishing Group, 1982.

Wigmore, Ann. *The Hippocrates Diet and Health Program*. U.S.: Avery Publishing Group, 1984.

Wills, Judith. *The Omega Diet*. London: Headline, 2002.

Wilson, Dr. Robert C. D. *Pre-Menstrual Syndrome: Diet Against It*. Berkshire: Foulsham, 1989.

Wilson, Frank Avray. *Food Fit for Humans*. U.K.: The C. W. Daniel Company, 1975.

Yiamouyiannis, Dr. John. *Fluoride: The Aging Factor*. U.S.: Health Action Press, 1993.

Yiamouyiannis, John. *High Performance Health*. U.S.: Health Action Press, 1987.

Youngson, Dr. Robert. *The Antioxidant Health Plan*. U.K.: Thorsons, 1994.

Yudkin, John. *This Slimming Business*. Middlesex: Penguin, 1974.

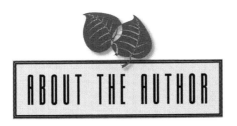

ABOUT THE AUTHOR

PLAGUED FOR MANY YEARS by ill health, Mary-Ann Shearer embarked on a personal quest for a common-sense approach to health and well-being. Her intensive studies into nutrition and a natural lifestyle over nearly thirty years led her to develop a simple yet highly effective program that produced unimagined levels of health and vitality. The first to benefit were her family and friends, but after several years of one-on-one consultations, she wrote the book *The Natural Way: A Family's Guide to Vibrant Health* (now in its twenty-first reprint) to help meet the growing demand for her time and knowledge. Since then, Mary-Ann has helped many thousands of people to understand and correct their diet-related problems, thereby building a valuable database of case studies that backs her ongoing research.

Mary-Ann has also published two recipe books (*The Natural Way: Recipe Book 1* and *The Natural Way: Recipe Book 2*), each a compilation of more than 300 recipes developed during her popular cooking demonstrations. Her books have been run-away bestsellers, outperforming all other natural health titles in southern Africa. *Healthy Kids: The Natural Way* was released at the end of 2001 to wide acclaim. *Perfect Weight: The Natural Way* was released in August 2003 and has had record sales to date. *Take Control,* written by both Mark and Mary-Ann Shearer, was released in May 2005 and is set to match the extraordinary sales records of its predecessors.

Further books are in the pipeline, including a full-color recipe book on healthy entertaining and a definitive reference work entitled *The A–Z of Natural Health.* Together with her husband, Mark, Mary-Ann runs seminars on "Finding the Balance," "Take Control," and "Sex, Drugs, and Cinnamon Rolls," subjects covered in detail in their book *Take Con-*

trol. She also contributes to numerous magazines and journals on an ongoing basis.

Mary-Ann has, over the years, addressed many diverse groups of people throughout the world, from farmers' wives in the heartland of South Africa, to professional medical people in Houston, Texas. She is in demand as a motivational speaker and regularly addresses groups at business seminars, schools, churches, and various associations such as the Cancer Association. She also appears frequently on national television and radio and had her own slot on national talk radio for many years.

Mary-Ann visits the U.K. and the U.S. regularly, where she is fast becoming a speaker in demand.

Technikon South Africa (now part of Unisa—one of the biggest correspondence universities in the world) has approved her Natural Health and Nutrition Course, and more than 650 students have enrolled worldwide.

Mary-Ann's aim is to show that it is fun and easy to be healthy, and it is this philosophy that inspires her many projects. She and her husband Mark have developed a unique range of whole food products for the retail market. They run their business from Stellenbosch in the Cape.

She sends out a regular free e-mail newsletter. Mark and Mary-Ann also film an entire three- to four-hour monthly Digimag, a digital magazine on DVD that can be ordered online or by fax. This service can be accessed on her Web site www.mary-anns.com.

47766294R00161

Made in the USA
San Bernardino, CA
11 April 2017